THE ROLE OF PLATELETS IN BLOOD-BIOMATERIAL INTERACTIONS

The Role of Platelets in Blood-Biomaterial Interactions

Edited by

Y.F. MISSIRLIS

and

J.-L. WAUTIER

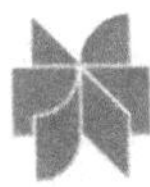

SPRINGER SCIENCE+BUSINESS MEDIA, B.V.

Library of Congress Cataloging-in-Publication Data

The Role of platelets in blood-biomaterial interactions / edited by
Y.F. Missirlis and J.-L. Wautier.
p. cm.
Includes bibliographical references and index.
ISBN 978-0-7923-2162-0 ISBN 978-94-011-1745-6 (eBook)
DOI 10.1007/978-94-011-1745-6
1. Biomaterials--Congresses. 2. Blood platelets--Aggregation--Congresses. 3. Biocompatibility--Congresses. I. Missirlis, Y. F., 1946- . II. Wautier, J.-L.
[DNLM: 1. Biocompatible Materials--congresses. 2. Blood Platelets--physiology--congresses. WH 300 R745 1993]
R857.M3R65 1993
610'.28--dc20
DNLM/DLC
for Library of Congress 93-2728

ISBN 978-0-7923-2162-0

Printed on acid-free paper

Table of Contents

PART THREE:
DISCUSSION CHAPTERS

Foreword

The present book relates to the scientific records of an expert meeting entitled "The Role of Platelets in Blood, Biomaterials Interactions" which was held in Pythagorion, Greece in May 1992, under the auspices and with financial support of the European Economic Communities (Concerted Action EUROBIOMAT – Hemocompatibility – of the Medical Research Programme, Project:II.1.2/2). This Concerted Action promotes the collaboration on science and technology on the particular field of hemocompatible biomaterials: exchange of experts, scholarships and scientific workshops within the EC-member countries and COST countries such as the Scandinavian countries, Turkey, Switzerland, Austria.

The first part of this monograph refers to the oral presentations of the participants. The second part gives the book its unique character: the scientific discussion on updated aspects of the properties and the behaviour of platelets. This second part is subdivided into six chapters where specific topics were discussed freely, open-minded and even controversially.

This book intends to elucidate recurrent questions concerning the properties of platelets and their behaviour when blood contacts artificial surfaces. Young investigators will consider this book to be appropriate to get familiar with the scientific background.

The international expert group of haematologists biochemists, polymer chemists and chemical engineers, exchanged ideas and arguments with respect to this interdisciplinary area, the interaction of thrombocytes at the interface of biomaterial surfaces.

W. Lemm

Acknowledgements

Apart from the participants who reworked meticulously their contribution to the discussion chapters I wish to thank especially the secretary of the Biomedical Engineering Laboratory, Mrs. Caterina Triantafyllopoulou for the overall contribution in preparing the Discussion chapters.

Y.F. Missirlis

List of Contributors

Dr. G. Athanassiou, Biomedical Engineering Laboratory, University of Patras, Rion, Patra 26100, Greece

Dr. C. Cerletti, Consorzio Mario Negri Sud, Centro di Riserche Farmacologiche e Biomediche, 66030 S. Maria Imbaro (Chieti), Italy

Dr. A. Davies, Academic Unit of Medicine, (Leeds General Infirmary), The University of Leeds, The Martin Wing, Leeds LS1 3EX, United Kingdom

Dr. St. Hanson, Division of Hematology-Oncology, Department of Medicine, Emory University, Woodruff Memorial Building, P.O. Box AR, Atlanta, GA 30322, U.S.A.

Dr. N. Kieffer, Laboratoire Franco-Luxembourgeois de Recherche Biomedical, Z.I. Grasbusch, L–3370 Leudelange, Luxembourg

Dr. W. Lemm, Rudolf-Virchow-Clinic, Charlottenburg, Spandauer Damm 130, D–1000 Berlin 19, Germany

Mr. G. Michanetzis, Biomedical Engineering Laboratory, University of Patras, Rion, Patras 26 100, Greece

Dr. Y.F. Missirlis, Biomedical Engineering Laboratory, University of Patras, Rion, Patras 26 100, Greece

Dr. J. Mulvihill, CRTS, 10 rue Spielmann, 67085 Strasbourg Cedex, France

Dr. A. Ordinas, Servicio Hemoterapia y Hemostasia, Hospital Clinic I Provincial, Villarroel, 170, 08036 Barcelona, Spain

Dr. J.-L. Wautier, Laboratoire Central d'Immunohematologie, Hopital Lariboisiere, 2, rue Ambroise-Pare, 75010 Paris, France

Preface

The platelets have been discovered more than 150 years ago but their modern history is tightly linked to the development of plastic surfaces. Glass tubes and pipets activate platelets; this fact did not allow for a comprehensive study of platelet physiology. The first progress was made by using siliconized pipets and tubes. The onset of plastic tubes corresponds to the expansion of the research on platelets. Simultaneously platelet transfusions which were very difficult and rare using siliconized glass bottles achieved an extraordinary development in the last 20 years due to the improvement of plastic bags.

The use of polymers for extracorporeal circulation, for biomaterials in general, pointed out the importance of the interaction of these materials with blood platelets. The introduction of prostheses used for vascular replacement or artificial heart has reinforced the interest for platelet biomaterial interaction.

The possibility to collect platelets in large amounts using an apheresis system and the need to store platelets for several days renewed the interest for understanding the mechanism of platelet interaction with hemocompatible surfaces. During the last years the increase of chemotherapy in cancer was associated with an increase in platelet transfusion support. During the same period more and more prosthetic devices have been introduced in human patients. Platelet biomaterial interaction is nowadays of high priority for Research and Development.

The meeting organized in Samos had a specific goal which was to put together experts of different areas dealing with platelets or biomaterials. It was impossible to collect all the results available on platelet-biomaterial-interaction, but most of the main topics were covered. The long discussions were an excellent opportunity to exchange informations but also to define the unanswered questions which are of importance for the future and the new direction of research.

We hope that the book will be a useful tool for the researchers working in that field but also for the executives who may find here some ideas of how to improve some aspects of the medical care on the technical but also on the economical point of view.

The interdisciplinarity of the workshop, the different countries represented in a spirit of open collaboration were an example of a meeting fruitful on the scientific but also on the human aspects.

Yannis F. Missirlis
Jean-Luc Wautier

PART ONE

Molecular basis for platelet interactions with biomaterials

1. Ultrastructure of platelets and platelet-surface interactions

A. ORDINAS, G. ESCOLAR

Servicio de Hemoterapia y Hemostasia, Hospital Clinic i Provincial, Barcelona, Spain

and

J.G. WHITE

Department of Laboratory Medicine and Pathology, Pediatrics, University of Minnesota, Minneapolis, USA

Ultrastructural features of platelets in suspension

Human platelets have a discoid form in their resting state. In order to relate structure to function, the anatomy of the platelet has been divided into several zones [1, 2]. The peripheral zone consists of membranes and closely associated structures providing the surface of the platelet and the walls of the channels making up the surface-connected open canalicular system (OCS) (Figure 1). An exterior coat or glycocalyx, rich in glycoproteins [3], provides the outermost covering of the peripheral zone. The middle layer of the peripheral zone is a typical unit membrane, rich in phospholipids, that serves as an essential surface for interaction with coagulation factors. Glycoproteins are embedded in the lipid bilayer of the unit membrane. They provide the receptors for stimuli triggering platelet activation. Heads of the glycoproteins extend to the extracellular space forming the glycocalyx. The tails are usually related to the submembrane zone and translate signals received on the outside surface into chemical messages and physical alterations required for platelet activation.

The sol-gel zone is the matrix of the platelet cytoplasm. It contains several fiber systems in various states of polymerization (cytoskeleton). These systems support the discoid shape in resting platelets and provide a contractile system involved in shape change, pseudopod extension, internal contraction and secretion. Elements of the contractile system constitute approximately 30–50 per cent of the total platelet protein.

The organelle zone consists of granules, electron dense bodies, peroxisomes, lysosomes, mitochondria, as well as discrete particles of glycogen randomly dispersed in the cytoplasm. It serves in metabolic processes and for the storage of enzymes, non-metabolic adenine nucleotides, serotonin, a variety of protein constituents and calcium.

Y. F. Missirlis and J.-L. Wautier (eds.), The Role of Platelets in Blood-Biomaterial Interactions, 3–13.

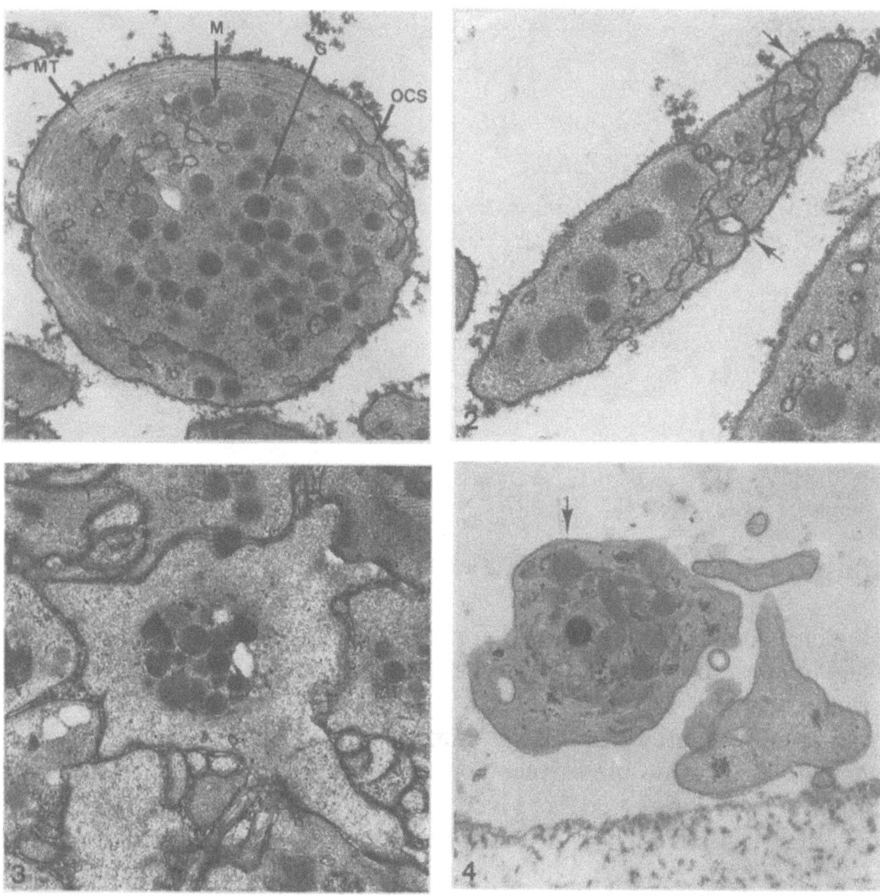

Figure 1–4. (1) Equatorial section of a discoid platelet. A circumferential microtubule band (MT) lying just under the surface membrane supports the discoid form. Granules (G), occasional mitochondria (M), and glycogen particles are irregularly distributed in the cytoplasm. Channels of the open canalicular system (OCS) and their conexion with the surface membrane have been made more evident by fixation in a tannic acid containing buffer. (17,280 ×) (2) Cross section of a discoid platelet stained with tannic acid. This mordant has facilitated the deposit of a darker coat that covers the exposed surface and evidences the connections of the surface membrane with the channels of the open canalicular system (arrows). (25,600 ×) (3) Platelets exposed to thrombin in suspension. The cell in the center has lost its discoid form, became irregular and developed internal transformation. Granules are concentrated in the center and enclosed within a constricted ring of microtubules. Elements of the open canalicular system (OCS) are filled with granule contents. Tannic acid osmium stained the material being released. During these processes platelets have interacted with each other forming an aggregate. (19,200 ×) (4) Platelet-vessel wall interaction. Endothelial cells were removed from rabbit aorta, the denuded segment inverted and exposed to flowing blood while placed in the rod of a Baumgartner chamber. Blood was maintained for 3 min at a shear rate of 800 sec^{-1}. Two cells have established contact with the subendothelium. One of them reveals early signs of activation (arrow). Organelles, including granules and a dense body are concentrated and enclosed by microtubules. (19,200 ×)

Membrane systems play a major role in platelet physiology. The dense tubular system (DTS) has been shown to be the site were calcium – important for triggering contractile events – is sequestered. The DTS is also the site where enzymes involved in prostaglandin synthesis are localized. The surface connected open canalicular system (OCS) provides access to the interior for plasma borne substances and a channel for products of the release reaction (Figure 2). Together with elements of the DTS, channels of the OCS form specialized membrane complexes which closely resemble the relationships of transverse tubules and sarcotubules in embryonic muscle cells.

Platelets are contractile blood elements with a specialized functional activity in hemostasis. The fundamental mechanisms of platelet function involve: adhesion (aggregation), contraction, and secretion. Platelets respond to a variety of chemical, particulate, and other stimuli in a characteristic manner [4–6]. The cells quickly lose their discoid shape, become relatively spherical in form, and extend long, spiky pseudopods, as well as bulky surface protrusions (Figure 3). Changes in the surface contour are accompanied by movement of randomly dispersed organelles toward the platelet centers. The transfer of granules and dense bodies is associated with constriction of the circumferential band of microtubules and contraction of the filamentous matrix of the sol-gel zone. Membranes of the α-granules fuse with those of the OCS thus facilitating the release of their content. As contents of the secretory organelles are extruded, the web of tubules and filaments continues to contract until only a mass of contractile gel remains in the central zone.

Ultrastructure of platelets interacting with vascular surfaces

Studies in animal models have demonstrated that platelets interact with sites experimentally denuded of endothelial cells. Several studies [7, 8] have shown that within the first minute, platelets interact with the exposed subendothelial surface. A continuous layer of platelets usually covers the damaged area within 20 min. The presence of mural platelet thrombi reaches its maximum after 10 min and disappear within 40 min.

Sequential studies in the perfusion system developed by Baumgartner have provided information on the morphology of platelet interacting with vascular surfaces [7]. Platelets first interact with the subendothelial elements usually through one or two pseudopods. At this initial stage platelets may still retain their discoid shape or show early signs of activation (Figure 4). In a more advanced stage platelets spread on the surface in an attempt to cover the denuded subendothelium. In the next seconds and depending on the flow conditions, more platelets will be recruited on the initially established monolayer which will lead to the formation of aggregates (Figure 5).

The perfusion system originally developed by Baumgartner [7] has contributed to the understanding of the specific mechanisms involved in platelet adhesion to vascular components. In this system, vascular surfaces of dif-

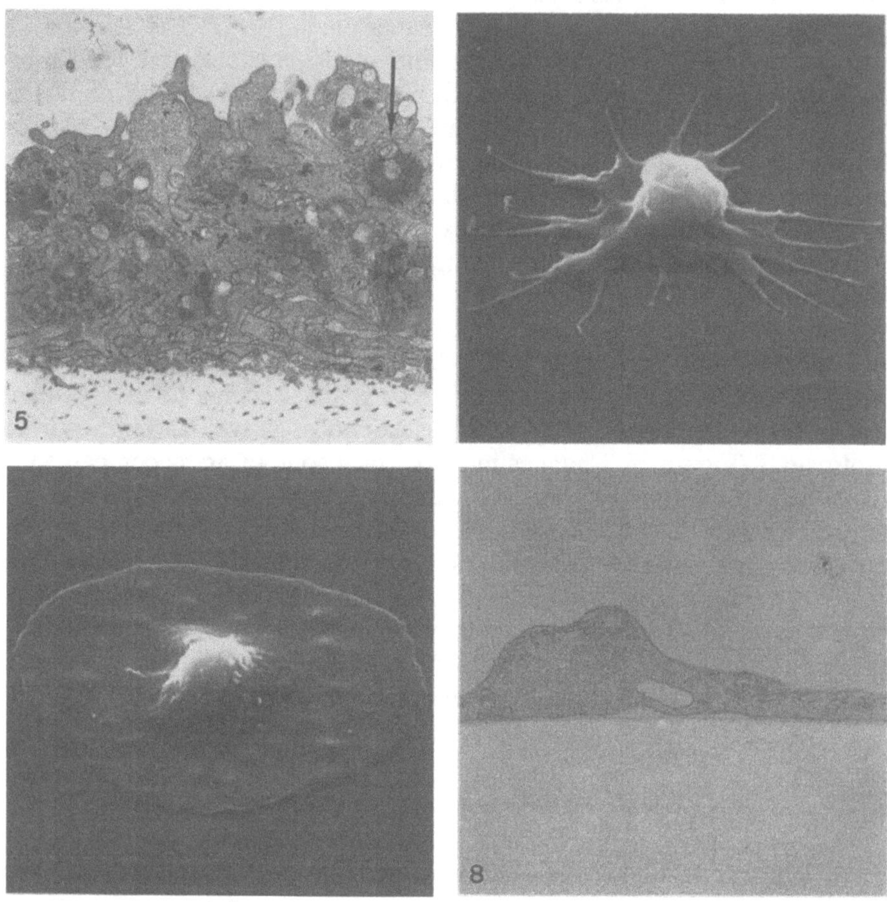

Figure 5–8. (5) Platelet-vessel wall interaction. After 10 min platelets from flowing blood have formed an aggregate on the denuded vessel segment. An initial layer of platelets have spread on the subendothelial cells. Other platelets have interacted with those previously spread. Interactions between aggregated platelets appears identical to those occurring in cells stimulated in suspension, including the process of internal transformation (arrow). (6,400 ×) (6) Platelet-artificial surface interaction. Platelet from a drop of citrated platelet rich plasma allowed to interact with a carbon-coated polymer surface for 20 min. The cell has lost its discoid shape and becomes relatively spherical. Portions of the surface in contact with the surface have extended long pseudopods. This is a typical dendritic form. (7,680 ×) (7) Platelet-artificial surface interaction. Interaction with the surface has caused this cell to spread into a thin film. centrally concentrated organelles protrude in the cell center. (7,680 ×) (8) Cross section of a platelet that has interacted with a polymer surface. This platelet has spread on the artificial surface. The open canalicular system is apparent. Alpha granules are no longer visible in this cell. (12,800 ×)

ferent origins are exposed to circulating blood under defined flow conditions. Standardized studies performed in perfusion systems have facilitated the understanding of the basic roles of membrane glycoproteins in adhesion and aggregation of platelets onto damaged vessel wall. The binding of von Willebrand factor (vWF) to subendothelium and to platelet GPIb is of critical importance for platelet attachment to subendothelial components [9–11]. Subsequent platelet spreading and aggregate formation seem to be mediated by platelet GPIIb–IIIa [12, 13]. Interactions of platelet GPIIb–IIIa mediated by fibrinogen seem of special interest since this mechanism is basic for aggregate formation [12] and would be directly implicated in thrombotic complications.

While the physiological role of major platelet glycoproteins in mediating platelets interactions with denuded vascular surfaces is well established, it is uncertain that the same mechanisms and sequence of events are implicated in thrombosis on biomaterial surfaces.

Ultrastructure of platelets interacting with foreign surfaces

Under static conditions platelets interact with foreign surfaces, including glass and plastic polymers. This type of interaction does not require the presence of plasma proteins and, though it may be delayed, is not inhibited by antibodies against the most significant glycoproteins (GPIb and GPIIb–IIIa). Interactions of platelets with foreign surfaces result in changes similar to those observed in suspended cells following activation. The cells become irregular and extend pseudopods in many directions (Figure 6). In more advanced stages, spaces between pseudopods are filled in, resulting in an appearance resembling a fried egg (Figure 7). The surface of the platelet away from the elevated central area is smooth and featureless. Platelets interacting with surfaces develop the same internal transformations as cells activated in suspension (Figure 8). Concentration of organelles in the center of cells and release of alpha granules can be identified in cross sections.

Although morphology appears similar to that described for platelets interacting with subendothelial surfaces. The series of events that result in platelet surface activation do not have to be the same. As already mentioned plasma proteins are not required for platelets to interact with polymer surfaces under static conditions. However, plasma proteins play a critical role in facilitating interactions of platelets under *in vivo* situations. Early studies demonstrated that absorption of plasma proteins on biomaterials is the initial event leading to thromboembolic complications [14–16]. Studies in different experimental models involving different animal species have documented that absorption of fibrinogen, fibronectin or von Willebrand factor on polymer surfaces influence the deposition of platelets [17, 18]. At present, it is well established that a thin layer of plasma proteins is deposited on artificial surfaces within seconds after they are exposed to blood. There is reasonable evidence indicating that the composition of this protein film determines the thrombogenic properties of the polymer surfaces [19, 20]. Although, different adhesive proteins of the plasma are involved, fibrinogen seems to play a major role in this thrombogenic process [15, 16, 19, 21–23]. Recent work has provided evidence that fibrinogen undergoes conformational changes after adsorption on polymer surfaces [24]. It has been suggested that non-stimulated platelets may attach to immobilized fibrinogen through interactions of the GPIIb–IIIa complex. This initial attachment would be independent of platelet activation, could be followed by irreversible adhesion and would not be interfered with by inhibitors of platelet function [25].

Localization of GPIb and GPIIb–IIIa receptors on platelets interacting with foreign surfaces: Do fibrinogen receptors move?

Two specialized areas of interaction can be distinguished in platelets that have interacted with a surface. The abluminal or ventral side with which platelets relate to the substrata and the luminal or dorsal side that provides a relation of the attached platelet with other platelets or cell elements. The dorsal side is an interface of critical importance for the development of thrombosis. Arrangement and interactions of receptors with specific ligands would allow other platelets to be recruited on the initial layer of platelets to constitute larger aggregates. A series of recent investigations have used formvar films to investigate the organization of fibrinogen receptor after surface activation of human platelets [26–29]. The size and thickness of platelets during spreading on formvar films have enormously facilitated their study "en face" in the electron microscope. Investigations in these systems using colloidal gold markers have provided new insights on the specific changes taking place on the luminal side of platelets activated by polymer surfaces. Studies performed with fibrinogen coupled to colloidal gold particles [26, 30, 31] demonstrated the expression of fibrinogen receptors on surface activated platelets.

In their study Loftus and Albrecht [26] suggested that receptors for fibrinogen expressed on GPIIb–IIIa underwent spontaneous reorganization. This initial work emphasized the fact that Fgn-Au complexes were moved from peripheral margins toward centers of surface activated platelets. Though these observations have been confirmed by studies in our laboratories [27, 32–35], the more recent evidence indicates that Fgn-Au bound to receptors seldom reached the central zone (Figure 9). Instead, they entered channels of the surface-connected open canalicular system (OCS) in over 40% of dendritic platelets and 5% to 15% of fully spread platelets [27, 32, 36]. Further studies have demonstrated that centralization of Fgn-Au loaded receptors can be achieved after washing the grids for a few minutes on buffer solutions (Figure 10).

Studies in which platelets interacting with formvar surfaces were fixed after spreading (Figure 11) showed that immunogold labelling of GPII–IIIa revealed edge-to-edge localization of this receptors [37]. The latter results

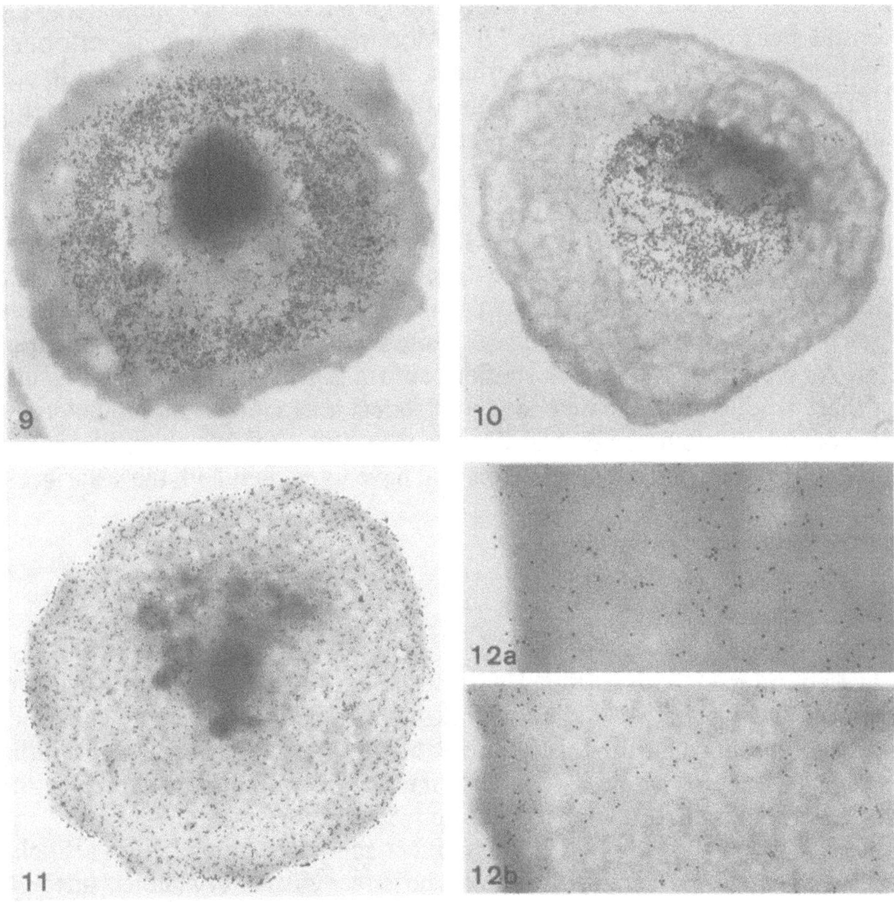

Figure 9–12. (9) Fully spread platelet allowed to interact with a carbon coated polymer surface for 20 min and exposed to fibrinogen coupled to colloidal gold (Fgn-Au) for 5 min before fixation. Fgn-Au has moved from the peripheral zone to the intermediate zone. The central zone is relatively devoid of Fgn-Au receptor complexes.(4,100 ×) (10) This platelet has been basically prepared as in Figure 9 with the exception that it was washed and exposed to buffer solution before fixation. Centralization of fibrinogen receptors can be achieved under these conditions. (4,100 ×) (11) Platelet exposed to a carbon coated polymer surface and fixed in a low concentration of glutaraldehyde and then incubated with fibrinogen gold (Fgn-Au) for 5 min. Glycoprotein IIb–IIIa receptors labeled by Fgn-Au extend from one edge of the cell to the other. (4,100 ×) (12) Detail of spread platelets allowed to interact with a carbon coated polymer surface for 20 min and fixed. Glycoprotein Ib or glycoprotein IIb–IIIa were detected by incubation with specific monoclonal antibodies followed by exposure to the correspondent gold labelled secondary antibody: (a) Glycoprotein Ib appears randomly distributed on the dorsal surface of the platelet. (b) Glycoprotein IIb–IIIa was also localized on the dorsal surface of platelets but with an apparent increased frequency over cell margins. (32,000 ×)

showing random distribution of GPIIb–IIIa receptors in spread platelets seem in contradiction with the observations of Fgn-Au being concentrated into the central areas of spread platelets [26]. More recent investigations performed on platelets spread on formvar surfaces after immunolabelling for GPIb and GPIIb–IIIa have confirmed that both GPIb and GPIIb–IIIa are present on the dorsal surface of spread platelets. The morphological analysis of these preparations revealed that GPIIb–IIIa complexes were distributed edge to edge in fixed spread platelets, and were more densely located over the marginal portions of spread cells (Figure 12). All these data suggest that fgn receptors probably do not undergo spontaneous reorganization during the shape changes involved in surface activation. It is very likely that the particulate (gold) but not fibrinogen is the real stimulus that triggers the movement of Fgn-Au particles [37]. Recent studies confirm this hypothesis [28]. If results of these studies are to be extended to platelets interacting with biomaterials, the conclusion would be that GPIIb–IIIa receptors – ready to bind fibrinogen – are likely to be present on platelets that have interacted with these surfaces.

Summary

Platelets interact with artificial surfaces. Shortly after exposure to a foreign surface, platelets become sticky. Almost immediately, they extend pseudopods adopting dentritic forms. Subsequently, the cytoplasm expands filling spaces between pseudopods. Platelets interacting with surfaces develop the same internal transformation as cells activated in suspension.

The mechanisms implied in the initial attachment of platelets on artificial surfaces, such as polymers, differ from those recognized for platelets interacting with vascular surfaces. An early deposition of plasma adhesive proteins seem to play a fundamental role in initiating platelet surface interactions. Despite their limitations, studies on platelets interacting with formvar coated grids have provided a unique model to analyze in detail changes taking place at the luminal face of surface activated platelets. The dorsal surface of spread platelets constitutes the critical interface where thrombotic complications will be initiated.

Most of the strategies to prevent thrombotic complications on biomaterials have focussed on the avoidance of protein and initial platelet deposition on polymers. Results of these strategies have not been dramatically successful. The initial attachment of platelets on polymers is difficult to prevent. The more recent evidence suggests that platelets possess several receptors that can be used to mediate attachment through interactions with different domains expressed on adhesive proteins. GPIIb–IIIa remains the basic receptor mediating platelet-platelet interactions. If a message is to be learned from the present review it would be that platelets interacting with surfaces express GPIb and fibrinogen receptors on their dorsal surface. Expression of the latter receptor is likely to support the recruitment of platelets to form larger aggregates.

Studies in experimental models of thrombosis have repeatedly demonstrated that formation of platelet aggregates on denuded arteries is self-limited. After a certain period of time aggregates disappear and monolayers of platelets refractory to other circulating platelets remain at injury sites. New approaches should be considered to prevent thrombotic complications on biomaterials. It is possible that less interference with the early attachment of platelets on polymer surfaces, but more specific intervention to avoid platelet-platelet interaction would result in a more effective prevention of thrombotic complications. New antiplatelet agents, including monoclonal antibodies against conformational changes in receptor or ligand binding sites and specific peptides, are available. These strategies may ultimately prove to be more successful than current methods in limiting thrombosis on biomaterials.

Acknowledgements

Authors want to thank Marcy Krumwiede for the excellent technical assistance. This work was partially supported by grants: CIRIT EE87, FIS 1070/88, FIS 4146/90, DGICYT PM89/104, NIH–HL11880, NIH–GM22167 and MOD 1–886.

References

1. White, J. G., 'An overview of platelet structural physiology', *Scanning Microsc.* 1987, 1: 1677–700.
2. White, J. G., 'Platelet structural physiology: the ultrastructure of adhesion, secretion, and aggregation in arterial thrombosis', *Cardiovasc. Clin.* 1987, 18: 13–33.
3. Polley, M. J., Leung, L. L. K., Clark, F., and Nachman, R. L., 'Thrombin induced platelet membrane glycoprotein IIb and IIIa complex formation: An electron microscope study', *J. Exp. Med.* 1981, 154: 1058–1068.
4. White, J. G., 'Fine structural alterations induced in platelets by adenosine diphosphate', *Blood* 1968, 31: 604–622.
5. White, J. G. and Clawson, C. C., 'Overview article: biostructure of blood platelets', *Ultrastruct. Pathol.* 1980, 1: 533–558 ULTRAS.
6. White, J. G., 'The morphology of platelet function', *Meth. Hematol.* 1983, 4: 1–25.
7. Baumgartner, H. R., 'The role of blood flow in platelet adhesion, fibrin deposition and formation of mural thrombi', *Microvasc. Res.* 1973, 5: 167–179.
8. Turitto, V. T. and Baumgartner, H. R., 'Platelet adhesion', *Meth. Hematol.* 1983, 8: 46–63.
9. Bolhuis, P. A., Sakariassen, K. S., Sander, H. J., Bouma, B. N., and Sixma, J. J., 'Binding of factor VIII-von Willebrand factor to human arterial subendothelium precedes increased platelet adhesion and enhances platelet spreading', *J. Lab. Clin. Med.* 1981, 97: 568–576.
10. Turitto, V. T., Weiss, H. J., and Baumgartner, H. R., 'Decreased platelet adhesion on vessel segments in von Willebrand's disease: a defect in initial platelet attachment', *J. Lab. Clin. Med.* 1983, 102: 551–564.
11. Stel, H. V., Sakariassen, K. S., de Groot, P. G., van Mourik, J. A., and Sixma, J. J., 'Von Willebrand factor in the vessel wall mediates platelet adherence', *Blood* 1985, 65: 85–90.

12. Weiss, H. J., Turitto, V. T., and Baumgartner, H. R., 'Platelet adhesion and thrombus formation on subendothelium in platelets deficient in glycoproteins IIb–IIIa, Ib, and storage granules', *Blood* 1986, 67: 322–330.
13. Weiss, H. J., Turitto, V. T., and Baumgartner, H. R., 'Further evidence that glycoprotein IIb–IIIa mediates platelet spreading on subendothelium', *Thromb. Haemost.* 1991, 65: 202–205.
14. Baier, R. E. and Dutton, R. C., 'Initial events in interaction of blood with a foreign surface', *J. Biomed. Mater. Res.* 1969, 3: 191–206.
15. Zucker, M. B. and Vroman, L., 'Platelet adhesion induced by fibrinogen adsorbed onto glass', *Proc. Soc. Exp. Biol. Med.* 1969, 131: 318–320.
16. Vroman, L., Adams, A., Klings, M., and Fischer, G., 'Fibrinogen, globulins, albumin and plasma at interfaces', *Adv. Chem. Ser.* 1975, 145: 255–289.
17. Collins, W. E., Mosher, D. F., Diwan, A. R., Murthy, K. D., Scott, R. S., Albrecht, R. M., and Cooper, S. L., 'Ex vivo platelet deposition on fibronectin-preabsorbed surfaces', *Scanning Microsc.* 1987, 1: 1669–1676.
18. Lambrecht, L. K., Young, B. R., Stafford, R. E., Park, K., Albrecht, R. M., Mosher, D. F., and Cooper, S. L., 'The influence of preabsorbed canine von Willebrand factor, fibronectin and fibrinogen on ex vivo artificial surface-induced thrombosis', *Thromb. Res.* 1986, 41: 99–117.
19. Feuerstein, I. A., Mcclung, W. G., and Horbett, T. A., 'Platelet Adherence and detachment with adsorbed fibrinogen – a flow study with a series of hydroxyethyl-methacrylate ethyl-methacrylate copolymers using video microscopy', *J. Biomed. Mater. Res.* 1992, 26: 221–237.
20. Kishida, A., Mishima, K., Corretge, E., Konishi, H., and Ikada, Y., 'Interactions of poly(ethylene glycol)-grafted cellulose membranes with proteins and platelets', *Biomaterials* 1992, 13: 113–118.
21. Brash, J. L. and Davidson, J. V., 'Adsorption on glass and polyethylene from solutions of fibrinogen and albumin', *Thromb. Res.* 1976, 9: 249–259.
22. Park, K., Mosher, D. F., and Cooper, S. L., 'Acute surface-induced thrombosis in the canine ex vivo model: Importance of protein composition of the initial monolayer and platelet activation', *J. Biomed. Mater. Res.* 1986, 20: 589–612.
23. Chinn, J. A., Horbett, T. A., and Ratner, B. D., 'Baboon fibrinogen adsorption and platelet adhesion to polymeric materials', *Thromb. Haemostas* 1991, 65: 608–617.
24. Shiba, E., Lindon, J. N., Kushner, L., Matsueda, G. R., Hawiger, J., Kloczewiak, M., Kudryk, B., and Salzman, E. W., 'Antibody-detectable changes in fibrinogen adsorption affecting platelet activation on polymer surfaces', *Am. J. Physiol.* 1991, 260: C965–C974.
25. Savage, B. and Ruggeri, Z. M., 'Selective recognition of adhesive sites in surface-bound fibrinogen by glycoprotein-IIb–IIIa on nonactivated platelets', *J. Biol. Chem.* 1991, 266: 11227–11233.
26. Loftus, J. C. and Albrecht, R. M., 'Redistribution of the fibrinogen receptor of human platelets after surface activation', *J. Cell. Biol.* 1984, 99: 822–829.
27. Leistikow, E. A., Barnhart, M. I., Escolar, G., and White, J. G., 'Receptor-ligand complexes are cleared to the open canalicular system of surface-activated platelets', *Br. J. Haematol.* 1990, 74: 93–100.
28. Estry, D. W., Mattson, J. C., Mahoney, G. J., and Oesterle, J. R., 'A comparison of the fibrinogen receptor distribution on adherent platelets using both soluble fibrinogen and fibrinogen immobilized on gold beads', *Eur. J. Cell. Biol.* 1991, 54: 196–210.
29. Kieffer, N., Guichard, J., and Breton-Gorius, J., 'Dynamic redistribution of major platelet surface receptors after contact-induced platelet activation and spreading – an immunoelectron microscopy study', *Am. J. Pathol.* 1992, 140: 57–73.
30. Goodman, S. L. and Albrecht, R. M., 'Correlative light and electron microscopy of platelet adhesion and fibrinogen receptor expression using colloidal-gold labelling', *Scanning Microsc.* 1987, 1: 727–734.
31. Oliver, J. A. and Albrecht, R. M., 'Colloidal gold labeling of fibrinogen receptors in

epinephrine and ADP-activated platelet suspensions', *Scanning Microsc.* 1987, 1: 745–756.

32. Escolar, G., Leistikow, E., and White, J. G., 'The fate of the open canalicular system in surface and suspension-activated platelets', *Blood* 1989, 74: 1983–1988.
33. White, J. G., Leistikow, E. L., and Escolar, G., 'Platelet membrane responses to surface and suspension activation', *Blood Cells* 1990, 16: 43–72.
34. White, J. G. and Escolar, G., 'Induction of receptor clustering, patching, and capping on surface-activated platelets', *Lab. Invest.* 1990, 63: 332–340.
35. White, J. G. and Escolar, G., 'Mobility of GPIIb–IIIa receptors within membranes of surface- and suspension-activated platelets does not depend on assembly and contraction of cytoplasmic actin', *Eur. J. Cell. Biol.* 1990, 52: 341–348.
36. Escolar, G. and White, J. G., 'The platelet open canalicular system: A final common pathway', *Blood Cells* 1991, 17: 467–485.
37. White, J. G. and Escolar, G., 'Fibrinogen receptors do not undergo spontaneous redistribution on surface-activated platelets', *Arteriosclerosis* 1990, 10: 738–744.

2. Structure and function of platelet membrane glycoproteins

N. KIEFFER

French-Luxembourg Biomedical Research Laboratory, Z.I. Grasbusch, L–3370 Leudelange, Luxembourg

Introduction

Platelets are involved in a variety of cellular interactions that occur during the hemostatic and inflammatory responses to tissue injury. These include adhesion to extracellular matrix proteins (e.g. von Willebrand factor, collagen, fibronectin, vitronectin, laminin), homotypic interaction with each other to form a platelet plug, and heterotypic interaction with other cells of the vasculature to promote the inflammatory response. Because platelet functions depend primarily on adhesive interactions, it is not too surprising that most of the glycoproteins on the platelet membrane surface are receptors for adhesive proteins or otherwise mediate cellular interactions. Many of these receptors have been identified: most have been cloned and sequenced and can now be classified within larger gene families of cell adhesion molecules which mediate a wide variety of cellular interactions. There are currently four known gene families of cell adhesion molecules. These include the Ca^{2+} dependent cadherins, the Ca^{2+} independent CAMs (cell adhesion molecules) of the immunoglobulin supergene family, the Ca^{2+} dependent selectins and the divalent cation dependent integrins (reviewed in Hynes and Lander, 1992). Interestingly, members of 3 of these gene families are present in platelets: integrins, CAMs and selectins. Platelets also express members of the leucine rich glycoprotein (LRG) gene family (reviewed in Roth, 1991). Although LRG members are not considered as typical cell adhesion molecules, in platelets they clearly function as such. Here I summarize recent information on the structure of platelet membrane glycoproteins, their relationship to larger gene families of cell adhesion molecules and their role in platelet functions.

Platelet membrane receptors of the leucine-rich glycoprotein gene family: The GPIb-V-IX system

The GPIb-IX complex

The GPIb-IX complex is the most prominent sialoglycoprotein of the platelet membrane (25,000 molecules per platelet) and contributes to the net negative

Y. F. Missirlis and J.-L. Wautier (eds.), The Role of Platelets in Blood-Biomaterial Interactions, 15–32.

charge of the platelet surface (reviewed in Clemetson, 1985; Roth, 1991). This complex consists of a large GPIbα chain (M_r = 143 000), a smaller disulfide linked GPIbβ chain (M_r = 22 000) and the non-covalently associated GPIX (M_r = 20 000). All 3 glycoproteins have been cloned (Lopez *et al.* 1987, 1988; Hickey *et al.* 1990) and belong to the leucine rich glycoprotein (LRG) gene family, sharing a common structural motif composed of a leucine-rich, 24 amino acid consensus sequence: P X X L L X X X X X L X X LX L S X N X L X X L (Takahashi *et al.* 1985). The GPIb-IX complex has an elongated, 60 nm in length dumbbell shape with a larger globular domain on one end used for membrane insertion and a smaller globular domain oriented external to the plasma membrane (Fox *et al.* 1988). Trypsin cleavage of the GPIb-IX complex releases the large extracellular domain of GPIbα, termed glycocalicin, leaving a membrane bound fragment of GPIbα of M_r = 25,000 disulphide-linked to GPIbβ and associated with GPIX (Du *et al.* 1987).

Receptor function

The major role of the GPIb-IX complex to platelet function is to bind to immobilized von Willebrand factor on exposed vascular subendothelium and thus initiate adhesion of platelets to the subendothelium at the site of vessel injury. This was established initially by the study of platelets from patients with Bernard Soulier syndrome, an inherited bleeding disorder (reviewed in George *et al.* 1984). Platelets from these individuals are defective in adhesion, do not bind von Willebrand factor and lack the GPIb-IX complex. In support of this function for GPIb, monoclonal antibodies directed against GPIbα also block adhesion of normal platelets to immobilized von Willebrand factor (Weiss *et al.* 1986). It is of interest that under normal flow conditions, GPIb does not bind soluble von Willebrand factor in plasma; apparently this protein undergoes a conformational change upon binding to the extracellular matrix which then exposes a recognition sequence for GPIb-IX (reviewed in Roth, 1991). The antibiotic ristocetin is most likely able to induce a similar change in the structure of soluble von Willebrand factor. The von Willebrand factor binding domain of the GPIb-IX complex has been narrowed down to a sequence encompassing amino acids 251 through 279 of GPIbα (Vincente *et al.* 1990). The GPIbα binding domain of von Willebrand factor resides in a tryptic fragment extending from residue 449 to 728 of the constituent subunit which does not contain an RGD sequence (Fujimura *et al.* 1986). This domain is formed by residues contained in two discontinuous sequences linked in the native molecule by disulfide binding (Mohri *et al.* 1989, Andrews *et al.* 1989). The GPIb-IX complex has also been reported to bind thrombin (Harmon & Jamieson 1986) as well as quinine/quinidine drug-dependent antibodies (Berndt *et al.* 1985).

The cytoplasmic domain of the GPIb-IX complex has a major function in linking the plasma membrane to the submembranous skeleton, a structure that in platelets is composed of short actin filaments linked to actin binding protein (ABP) and functions to stabilize the plasma membrane and maintain the discoid shape of the platelet (Fox *et al.* 1988). In resting platelets, the GPIb-IX complex interacts with the M_r = 540,000 dimeric actin binding protein. Upon platelet stimulation, this association is disrupted by an endogenous Ca^{2+}-dependent protease, which rapidly cleaves the M_r = 270,000 ABP subunit into three fragments (Ezzell *et al.* 1988). Interestingly, Bernard Soulier patients which lack GPIb-IX, are large, polymorphic cells, whose size and shape may be due to a lack of membrane-cytoskeleton association. When resting platelets are incubated with ^{32}P-phosphate, only the GPIbβ-subunit of the GPIb-IX complex becomes phosphorylated predominantly at serine residues and to a lesser extent at threonine residues (Wyler *et al.* 1986). Fox *et al.* (1987) have shown that phosphorylation of the β-chain of GPIb as well as ABP is increased under conditions that increase the concentration of cAMP, suggesting that the GPIb-IX complex may also be involved in regulating intracellular reactions in platelets by maintaining platelets in a resting state.

Glycoprotein V

GPV (M_r = 82,000) is another platelet membrane glycoprotein with multiple copies of the LRG motif (Schimomura *et al.* 1990; Roth *et al.* 1990). This glycoprotein, which is also deficient in patients with Bernard Soulier syndrome, has recently been shown to be associated with the GPIb-IX complex in platelet membranes (Modderman *et al.* 1992). GPV is unique in that it is the only major platelet membrane glycoprotein that is hydrolyzed by thrombin during platelet activation (Berndt & Phillips, 1981). When GPV is hydrolyzed, a water soluble fragment of GPV termed GPV_{fl} (M_r = 69,000) is released; the presumptive membrane-bound fragment has not yet been identified. The precise role of GPV in platelet function remains so far unclear.

Platelet membrane receptors of the integrin gene family

Integrins constitute a large family of related $\alpha\beta$ heterodimers which are widely distributed on many cells and are involved in cell-matrix or cell-cell interactions. There are currently about 20 known integrins, made up of various pairings of 8 distinct but homologous β-subunits and 20 α-subunits, each heterodimer having a distinct ligand specificity (Hynes, 1987; 1992). The common picture emerging from recent development in integrin research is that integrins may be divided into two major receptor groups, the activation-independent and the activation-dependent receptors. Integrins involved in cell-matrix interactions appear to belong to the first group, whereas integrins involved in cellular interactions are essentially members of the second group. Yet some integrins exhibit a dual receptor function as they mediate both cell-matrix and cell-cell interactions.

Platelets express 5 integrins which include, in order of decreasing amounts, glycoprotein IIb-IIIa ($\alpha_{IIb}\beta_3$), GPIa-IIa ($\alpha_2\beta_1$), GPIc-IIa ($\alpha_5\beta_1$), GPIc′-IIa ($\alpha_6\beta_1$) and the vitronectin receptor ($\alpha_v\beta_3$) (reviewed in Kieffer and Phillips, 1990). Platelet β_1 integrins, which are constitutively active receptors and are essentially involved in platelet adhesion to insoluble fibronectin ($\alpha_5\beta_1$), collagen ($\alpha_2\beta_1$) and laminin ($\alpha_6\beta_1$) present in the extracellular matrix, exhibit a highly restricted ligand specificity and recognize distinct recognition sequences within their respective ligands. In contrast, platelet β_3 integrins, GPIIb-IIIa ($\alpha_{IIb}\beta_3$) and the vitronectin receptor ($\alpha_v\beta_3$), are promiscuous receptors for a variety of soluble adhesive proteins found in plasma (fibrinogen, fibronectin, vitronectin, von Willebrand factor and thrombospondin) and recognize the tripeptide sequence Arg-Gly-Asp (RGD) in these ligands. The vitronectin receptor is constitutively active, whereas GPIIb-IIIa functions both as an activation-dependent and activation-independent receptor (Table 1).

GPIIb-IIIa

GPIIb-IIIa, which was the first well characterized member of the integrin gene family, serves as a prototype and is of particular interest, due to its major functional role in platelet aggregation. Normal platelets express about 50,000 molecules of GPIIb-IIIa on their surface. The GPIIb-IIIa complex is composed of one molecule of GPIIb (M_r = 140,000), which consists of a large α chain (M_r = 125,000) disulfide-linked to a light β chain (M_r = 22,000), and one molecule of GPIIIa (M_r = 150,000) which is a single poplypeptide chain. The GPIIb-IIIa complex is a Ca^{2+}-dependent heterodimer, noncovalently associated on the platelet surface (reviewed in Phillips *et al.* 1988). The mature GPIIIa polypeptide consists of 762 amino acids and contains a transmembrane domain and a cytoplasmic tail (Fitzgerald *et al.* 1987; Rosa *et al.* 1988). The extracellular domain consists of amino acid residues 1 through 692 and contains 56 cysteines, all of which are disulphide-linked (Calvete *et al.* 1991). The two chains of GPIIb are posttranslationally cleaved from a single precursor which remains disulfide linked (Bray *et al.* 1986). The large chain of mature GPIIb is formed of 871 amino acids and the light chain of 137 (Poncz *et al.* 1987). Only the light chain has a transmembrane domain. The large chain contains four repeating segments of about 65 amino acids each of which contains a 12 amino acid sequence characteristic of the Ca^{2+}-binding β turns of calmodulin. Ca^{2+} is required for maintenance of GPIIb and GPIIIa in the heterodimeric complex and for binding of adhesive proteins.

Receptor function

The critical functional role of GPIIb-IIIa in platelet aggregation was initially established by studies of platelets from patients with Glanzmann's thrombasthenia, an inherited bleeding disorder caused by a quantitative or qualitative defect of GPIIb-IIIa and a deficit of platelets to bind adhesive proteins and to aggregate (reviewed in George *et al.* 1990). Recent data suggest that GPIIb-IIIa might indeed exhibit a dual receptor function by mediating both

TABLE 1

Cell Adhesion Molecules Involved in Platelet Functions.

Glycoprotein	Receptor function	Ligand	Recognition sequence	Cation dependency
GPIIb-IIIa ($\alpha_{IIb}\beta_3$)	Activation dependent	Soluble Fb, Fn, Vn, vWF, TSP	RGD	Ca^{2+}
	Constitutive	Surface-bound Fb, Fibrin	HHLGGAKQAGD	Ca^{2+}
Vitronectin receptor ($\alpha_v\beta_3$)	Constitutive	Fb, Fn, Vn, vWF, TSP	RGD	Ca^{2+}
GPIa-IIa ($\alpha_2\beta_1$)	Constitutive	collagen	DGEA	Mg^{2+}
GPIc-IIa ($\alpha_5\beta_1$)	Constitutive	fibronectin	RGD	Ca^{2+}
GPIc′-IIa ($\alpha_6\beta_1$)	Constitutive	laminin	Elastase derived fragment E8	Mg^{2+}, Mn^{2+}
GMP-140 (P-selectin)	Constitutive	L-selectin ?	oligosaccharide Lewis^x (CD15)	Ca^{2+}
GPIIa (PECAM–1)	Constitutive	homophilic interaction	—	no
GPIV (IIIb)	?	TSP, collagen	?	Ca^{2+}

platelet aggregation and platelet adhesion. Also, GPIIb-IIIa appears to be a prototype of an integrin receptor whose adhesive specificity and affinity is posttranslationally regulated by conformational changes triggered by intracellular stimulus-response activation mechanisms as well as extracellular ligand occupancy.

Activation-dependent receptor function of GPIIb-IIIa during platelet aggregation. On resting circulating platelets, GPIIb-IIIa is surface exposed but does not interact with soluble ligands. Platelets are activated by a variety of agonists, such as thrombin, ADP, epinephrine, all of which act through seven transmembrane-helix receptors coupled to G proteins (reviewed in Manning and Brass, 1991). The stimulus-response coupled activation of GPIIb-IIIa through a primary receptor induces conformational changes in GPIIb-IIIa (Sims *et al.* 1991), leading to the exposure of high affinity binding sites for fibrinogen (inside-out signalling). These neo-epitopes can be monitored by certain GPIIb-IIIa monoclonal antibodies that bind to activated GPIIb-IIIa but not to resting GPIIb-IIIa (Shattil *et al.* 1985) (Figure 1A). Alternatively, some monoclonal antibodies, by binding to resting GPIIb-IIIa, are capable of inducing conformational changes of GPIIb-IIIa similar to those produced through stimulus-response coupled activation (Kouns *et al.* 1990; Gulino *et al.* 1990) (Figure 1B). Furthermore, chymotrypsin mediated proteolytic cleavage of membrane bound GPIIb-IIIa also induces the exposure of high affinity binding sites for fibrinogen with a concomitant release of a 3.7 KDa fragment of the carboxy-terminus of GPIIbα (Pidard *et al.* 1991). Athough the intracellular mechanism of the stimulus-response dependent activation process of GPIIb-IIIa in platelets is still unclear, recent data provide evidence that G proteins and activated protein kinase C are most likely involved (van Willigen & Akkermann, 1991; 1992).

The most potent plasma protein to mediate platelet aggregation is fibrinogen, although von Willebrand factor can also bind to GPIIb-IIIa and mediate platelet aggregation at high shear rates. Recent studies have characterized the molecular properties of ligand interaction with GP IIb-IIIa. The promiscuous capability of activated GPIIb-IIIa to interact with different adhesive proteins is due to its ability to bind to the RGD sequence contained within them. Although fibrinogen contains two RGD sequences in its α-chain, one near the N-terminus (residues 95–97) and a second near the C-terminus (residues 572–574) (Doolittle *et al.* 1979), immuno-inhibition experiments have shown that fibrinogen primarily uses the C-terminal RGD sequence to bind GPIIb-IIIa (Cheresh *et al.* 1989). A second site on fibrinogen that binds to GPIIb-IIIa has also been identified. This is the 12 amino acid sequence located at the carboxyl-terminus of the γ-chain of fibrinogen (Kloczewiak *et al.* 1989). This dodecapeptide is not found in other adhesive proteins, does not contain the RGD sequence, but competes with RGD-containing peptides for binding to GPIIb-IIIa (Lam *et al.* 1987). Peptides containing either RGD or dodecapeptide sequences inhibit the binding of fibrinogen, von Willebrand factor and fibronectin to the GPIIb-IIIa complex on activated platelets and therefore block platelet aggregation. Cross-linking studies of the RGD sequence to GPIIb-IIIa revealed that the peptide linked to GPIIIa 109–171 (D'Souza *et al.* 1988). In contrast, fibrinogen γ-chain dodecapeptide sequences cross-link to GPIIb 294–314 (D'Souza *et al.* 1990). A peptide from this region of GPIIb inhibits platelet aggregation and fibrinogen binding by interacting directly with fibrinogen (D'Souza *et al.* 1991). A third fibrinogen binding site has been localized to residues 211 through 222 of GPIIIa (Charo *et al.* 1989). Since RGD and the dodecapeptide interact with distinct sites on GPIIb-IIIa, their mutually competitive binding suggests that the binding of one sequence renders the second binding site nonfunctional. Although the mechanism how GPIIb-IIIa becomes activated is still unclear, O'Toole *et al.* (1991) have recently shown that truncation of the cytoplasmic part of GPIIbα increases the affinity of GPIIb-IIIa for fibrinogen, suggesting that this intracellular domain controls the receptor function of GPIIb-IIIa (Figure 1).

Activation-independent receptor function of GPIIb-IIIa during platelet adhesion. Resting GPIIb-IIIa in unactivated platelets is unable to bind soluble RGD containing adhesive proteins, however, GPIIb-IIIa on unstimulated platelets binds to immobilized fibrinogen, allowing for platelet adhesion to fibrinogen-coated surfaces. This activity of GPIIb-IIIa on unstimulated platelets differs from that of GPIIb-IIIa on stimulated platelets in that it is specific for fibrinogen with no binding to other RGD-containing adhesive proteins (Kieffer *et al.* 1991; Savage & Ruggeri, 1991). The receptor function of GPIIb-IIIa in nucleated cells is similar to that of GPIIb-IIIa in unstimulated platelets. In nucleated cells however, GPIIb-IIIa cannot be activated through a primary receptor dependent stimulus-response mechanism. Recent data provide evidence that one domain recognized by resting GPIIb-IIIa on surface-bound fibrinogen corresponds to the dodecapeptide sequence of the fibrinogen γ-chain (γ401–411)(Kieffer & Matsueda, 1991). As this domain is not recognized by resting GPIIb-IIIa on soluble fibrinogen, it is tempting to speculate that immobilization of fibrinogen, which induces conformational changes of the molecule similar to those observed after fibrinogen interaction with the receptor (neo-epitopes called RIBS, for "receptor-induced binding sites" on the ligand) (Zamarron *et al.* 1991), leads to the exposure of the dodecapeptide site, making it more easily accessible for resting GPIIb-IIIa interaction. Thus, resting GPIIb-IIIa interaction with immobilized fibrinogen might be a mechanism not only involved in circulating platelet adhesion to fibrin(ogen) and growing thrombi, but also in platelet aggregation (Figure 2), as well as heterotypic platelet interactions with other blood cells, such as activated leukocytes, recently shown to bind fibrinogen via β2 integrins (Altieri *et al.* 1990; Loike *et al.* 1991).

Receptor activation and signal transduction. It has been known for several years that the receptor function of GPIIb-IIIa is activated by stimulus-response

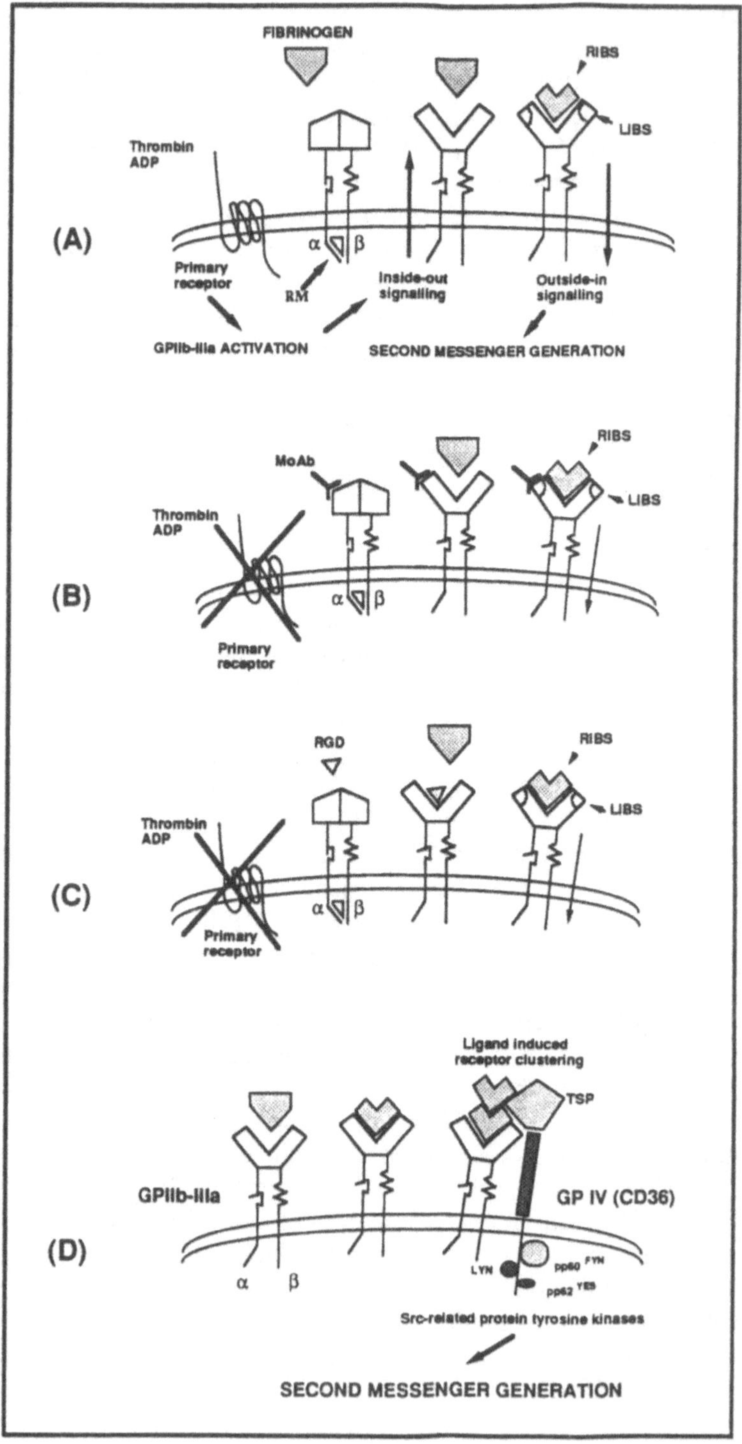
FIBRINOGEN
RIBS
LIBS
Thrombin
ADP
(A)
α
β
Primary
receptor
RM
Inside-out
signalling
Outside-in
signalling
GPIIb-IIIa ACTIVATION
SECOND MESSENGER GENERATION
MoAb
RIBS
LIBS
Thrombin
ADP
(B)
α
β
Primary
receptor
RGD
RIBS
LIBS
Thrombin
ADP
(C)
α
β
Primary
receptor
Ligand induced
receptor clustering
TSP
GPIIb-IIIa
GP IV (CD36)
(D)
α
β
LYN
pp60 FYN
pp62 YES
Src-related protein tyrosine kinases
SECOND MESSENGER GENERATION

← *Figure 1.* The figure summarizes data as well as hypotheses discussed in the texte concerning GPIIb-IIIa activation and GPIIb-IIIa mediated signal transduction during platelet aggregation. (A) Represented is a seven transmembrane helix receptor (thrombin receptor) and the $\alpha\beta$ integrin heterodimer GPIIb-IIIa under two distinct conformations: the closed conformation corresponding to the inactive receptor and the open conformation corresponding to the active receptor. GPIIb-IIIa on the surface of a resting platelet has a ligand-binding pocket but is not competent to bind the macromolecular ligand fibrinogen. Only after platelet activation by thrombin or other primary agonists does GPIIb-IIIa become an effective receptor for fibrinogen. Although the mechanism of the primary receptor-dependent activation of GPIIb-IIIa is still unknown, there is evidence that the cytoplasmic domain of GPIIb in some way is involved in a regulatory mechanism (RM) controlling the binding affinity of the extracellular domain of GPIIb-IIIa by maintaining it in a resting state. Activation of GPIIb-IIIa from inside the cell through the primary receptor is accompanied by conformational changes of both GPIIb and GPIIIa (inside-out signalling) leading to the exposure of high affinity binding sites for fibrinogen that can be monitored by monoclonal antibodies (shown is the activated receptor with an open fibrinogen binding pocket and a conformational change of the C-terminal part of GPIIbα). Fibrinogen, by binding to activated GPIIb-IIIa, induces further conformational changes and the expression of neoepitopes on GPIIb-IIIa, called 'LIBS' (for ligand induced binding sites). Bound fibrinogen itself undergoes conformational changes with the exposure of neoepitopes called 'RIBS' (for receptor induced binding sites). This ligand-receptor interaction and most likely receptor clustering finally leads to the activation of second-messenger pathways inside the platelet (outside-in signalling). (B) Some monoclonal antibodies, by binding to resting GPIIb-IIIa, are capable of inducing conformational changes of GPIIb-IIIa similar to those produced through stimulus-response coupled activation. (C) Small peptides derived from fibrinogen (RGDS, dodecapeptide γ401–411) bind to resting GPIIb-IIIa and directly activate the receptor leading to the exposure of secondary high affinity binding sites for fibrinogen. (D) Potential coclustering of GPIIb-IIIa with the thrombospondin receptor GPIV through fibrinogen – thrombospondin interaction. GPIV, which has protein tyrosine kinases associated with its cytoplasmic tail, might be involved in GPIIb-IIIa triggered tyrosine phosphorylation.

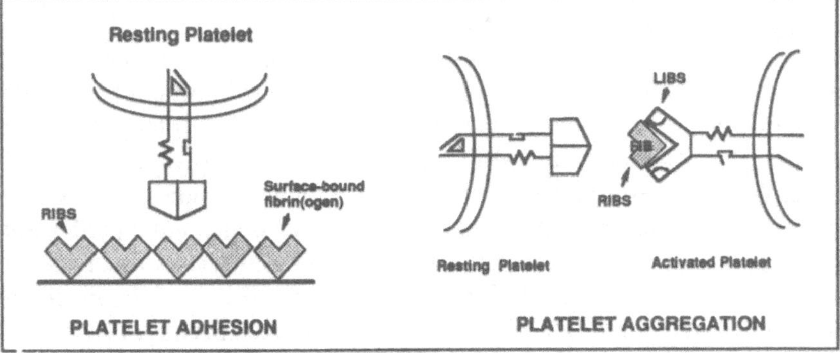

Figure 2. Potential functional role of resting GPIIb-IIIa in platelet adhesion and platelet aggregation.

mechanisms occurring during platelet activation. Recent data indicate that the binding of adhesive proteins to GPIIb-IIIa initiates additional events. RGD peptides and the dodecapeptide have been found to induce marked conformational changes with detergent solubilized GPIIb-IIIa (Parise *et al.* 1987). Furthermore, binding of RGD peptides to GPIIb-IIIa in resting platelets directly activates the receptor leading to the exposure on GPIIb-IIIa of secondary high affinity binding sites for fibrinogen (Du *et al.* 1991) (see Figure 1C). For GPIIb-IIIa in intact platelets, this change in conformation upon ligand binding can be demonstrated by the expression of neo-epitopes referred to as ligand-induced binding sites or "LIBS" (Frelinger *et al.* 1988; 1991) (see Figure 1A). These epitopes exist on both GPIIb and GPIIIa indicating that the conformation of both glycoproteins in the complex are affected by ligand occupancy. Other effects of ligand binding on GPIIb-IIIa include the de novo synthesis of metabolites of the phosphoinositide cascade such as PtdIns(3,4)P_2 (Sultan *et al.* 1991), an increase in tyrosine-specific protein phosphorylation (Ferrell & Martin, 1989; Golden *et al.* 1990), as well as an increase in Na^+/H^+ exchange in epinephrine-stimulated platelets (Banga *et al.* 1986). Ligand-receptor interactions also induce clustering of GPIIb-IIIa (Isenberg *et al.* 1986) or possibly clustering of GPIIb-IIIa with GPIV (see below and Figure 1D). Finally, ligand-receptor interaction leads to platelet aggregation, which additionally causes an increase in the phosphorylation of threonine residues of GPIIIa (Parise *et al.* 1990; Hillery *et al.* 1991) and the association of GPIIb-IIIa with the platelet cytoskeleton. Taken together, these data indicate that the conformational changes induced by the binding of adhesive proteins to GPIIb-IIIa are clearly involved in the generation of second messenger pathways.

The CD 36 antigen: Platelet glycoprotein IV

GPIV, also known as GPIIIb or CD36, is unique in that it has no sequence homology with any other known protein (Oquendo *et al.* 1989). It is a highly glycosylated 85 kDa glycoprotein, which is expressed in melanoma cells, monocytes, endothelial cells as well as nucleated erythroid cells, and which is distinguished by its high resistance to proteases in intact platelets (McGregor *et al.* 1989; Tandon *et al.* 1989). The role of GPIV in platelet function has not been definitely established. Several lines of evidence indicate that GPIV is a site for divalent cation-dependent binding of thrombospondin (TSP), and it has been proposed that TSP, which is a major α-granule protein secreted from platelets, serves as an extracellular bridge between GPIV and the fibrinogen-GPIIb-IIIa complex through TSP affinity for fibrinogen (Leung, 1984; Kieffer *et al.* 1988). Indeed, a monoclonal antibody to GPIV (OKM5) inhibits thrombospondin binding to thrombin activated platelets (Asch *et al.* 1987); purified GPIV binds to thrombospondin in a specific and Ca^{2+}-dependent manner and monospecific anti-GPIV antibodies partially inhibit thrombin-induced platelet aggregation (McGregor *et al.* 1989). The GPIV–thrombospondin interaction on platelets appears to occur as a two step process, with initial binding of thrombospondin to GPIV inducing a conformational change of thrombospondin and exposure of a second high affinity binding site for GPIV (Leung *et al.* 1991). More recently it has been shown that several src related tyrosine kinases are associated with GPIV in platelets (Huang *et al.* 1991), suggesting that either GPIV alone, or associated with GPIIb-IIIa in a multimeric complex might be involved in signal transduction. A role for GPIV as a collagen receptor has also been reported (Tandon *et al.* 1989). Nevertheless, the fact that GPIV is missing in platelets of 3–4% of healthy Japanese donors of the Nak^a phenotype having normal platelet functions questions the role of GPIV during platelet aggregation (Yamamoto *et al.* 1990).

The selectin gene family

The selectin gene family is a family of vascular cell surface receptors which are characterized by a lectin-like domain at their amino terminus, an adjacent epidermal growth factor-like domain, followed by multiple short consensus repeat units homologous to the complement regulatory proteins. There are currently three known selectins. One selectin is E-selectin (ELAM–1) whose expression is induced by cytokines on the surface of endothelial cells and functions as a receptor for neutrophils. Another has been termed L-selectin (LAM–1) essentially found on the cell surface of neutrophils and lymphocytes and functions in the homing of lymphocytes to specialized lymph node endothelium. P-selectin (GMP–140) is the only member of this family present in platelets (reviewed in McEver 1991).

P-selectin (Granule Membrane Protein 140, GMP–140)

P-selectin, also called GMP–140, PADGEM or CD62, is a 140 kDa integral membrane glycoprotein which contains nine complement binding repeats and is thus the largest selectin molecule, since E-selectin has six repeats and L-selectin only two (Johnston *et al.* 1989). P-selectin becomes exposed on the surface of activated platelets upon granule secretion. However, this exposure is transient since P-selectin expression decreases to background level within an hour after platelet activation, most likely due to receptor shedding or receptor endocytosis. P-selectin is also a constituent of endothelial cells where it is present in the membranes of Weibel Palade bodies and becomes exposed on the endothelial cell surface upon stimulation of the endothelium with inflammatory cytokines (reviewed in McEver, 1991).

Functional role of P-selectin in platelet interactions

Although P-selectin becomes exposed on the platelet surface following platelet activation, there is so far no clear evidence for P-selectin having an important functional role in platelet-platelet interactions. In contrast, P-selectin appears to be essentially involved in heterotypic platelet interactions with other cells. P-selectin functions as a receptor that mediates adherence of neutrophils and monocytes to activated platelets and endothelial cells (Larsen *et al.* 1989; Hamburger and McEver, 1990). This interaction is Ca^{2+}-dependent and can be inhibited by anti-P-selectin antibodies, purified P-selectin or selectin inserted in phospholipid vesicles. Recent data have provided evidence that P-selectin is a receptor for a specific carbohydrate structure, Lewis^x (CD15), which is attached to various glycoproteins and glycolipids present on the surface of neutrophils and monocytes (reviewed in Feizi, 1991). A possible functional role for P-selectin in platelet-leukocyte interactions might be to localize leukocytes to the site of vascular injury or alternatively, to localize platelets to the site of an inflammatory process. P-selectin might also function as a recognition system for macrophages to remove activated platelets from the circulating blood.

The immunoglobulin gene superfamily

The immunoglobulin gene superfamily is composed of several subfamilies of glycoproteins which are essentially involved in cellular recognition mechanisms and which all share a common structure called the immunoglobulin homology unit. Members of the immunoglobulin gene superfamily in platelets include HLA class I molecules, the Fcγ receptor as well as the CAM-related PECAM–1.

PECAM–1

The "platelet-endothelial cell adhesion molecule–1" (PECAM–1) (Newman *et al.* 1990) is a 130 kDa glycoprotein which was initially termed GPIIa on platelets and endothelial cells (van Mourik *et al.* 1985) and the leukocyte differentiation antigen CD31 on blood monocytes, neutrophils and mitogen-induced lymphoblasts (see Knapp *et al.* 1989). The cDNA deduced primary structure of PECAM–1 predicts an N-terminal extracellular domain of 574 amino acids with nine potential asparagine-linked glycosylation sites, a 19 residue transmembrane domain and a 118 residue cytoplasmic tail. The extracellular domain contains 12 cysteine residues that are spaced approximately 50 amino acids apart and flanked by six immunoglobulin-like homology units. The cytoplasmic domain of PECAM–1 contains a tyrosine that could serve as a phosphorylation site for tyrosine kinase. The structural homology of PECAM–1 to other CAM family members such as N-CAM and ICAM–1 and its localization in endothelial cells at the intercellular junctions supports the idea that PECAM–1 is essentially involved in homotypic cell interactions. Although PECAM–1 becomes rapidly phosphorylated after platelet stimulation by thrombin, its precise functional role in platelets is still unknown (Zehnder *et al.* 1992).

Other platelet membrane glycoproteins

A variey of minor platelet membrane glycoproteins have been identified whose structural properties and functional roles are still under investigation. Recently however, GPVI and a glycoprotein of 85–90 kDa have been implicated as additional collagen receptors based on the fact that platelets of a patient with GPVI deficiency failed to react to collagen (Moroi *et al.* 1989), and that an antibody against an 85–90 kDa glycoprotein in the plasma of a patient with prolonged bleeding time disturbed platelet aggregation to collagen (Deckmyn *et al.* 1992).

Summary and conclusion

The understanding of the structure and function of platelet membrane glycoproteins has been facilitated by studies showing that they belong to larger gene families of cell surface receptors involved in cellular interactions. In some instances, e.g. GPIIb-IIIa, the study of the platelet proteins has served as prototypes for relatively newly described gene families (integrins). In other instances, e.g. PECAM–1, the background of information on immunoglobulin domain containing proteins has served to indicate functions. For some platelet glycoproteins, receptor-ligand interactions have been characterized at the molecular level, and it becomes now apparent that the specificity and the affinity of these receptors and ligands are regulated or modulated posttranslationally through very subtle conformational changes. The precise knowledge of receptor-ligand interactions may lead to potential medical applications, such as the design of therapeutic analogues that will specifically inhibit aberrant pathological interactions of platelets during thrombotic or inflammatory responses to tissue injury.

Acknowledgement

This work was supported by grants from CRP–Santé, CNRS, Fondation de Recherche Cancer et Sang, and Fondation Alphonse Weicker, Luxembourg.

References

1. Altieri, D., Agbanyo, F., Plescia, J., Ginsberg, M., Edgington, T., and Plow, E., 'A unique recognition site mediates the interaction of fibrinogen with leukocyte integrin Mac1 (CD 11b/CD18)', *J. Biol. Chem.* 1991, 265: 12119–12122.
2. Andrews, R. K., Gorman, J. J., Booth, W. J., Corino, G. L., Castaldi, P. A., and Berndt, M. C., 'Cross-linking of a monomeric 39/34–kDa fragment of von Willebrand factor (leu-480/val–481-gly–781) to the N-terminal region of the α chain of membrane glycoprotein

Ib on intact platelets with bis (sulfosuccinimidyl) substrate', *Biochemistry* 1989, 28: 8326–8336.

3. Asch, A. S., Barnwell, J., Silverstein, R. L., and Nachman, R. L., 'Isolation of the thrombospondin membrane receptor', *J. Clin. Invest.* 1987, 79: 1054–1061.
4. Banga, H. S., Simons, E. R., Brass, L. F., and Rittenhouse, S. E., 'Activation of phospholipase A and C in human platelets exposed to epinephrine. Role of glycoproteins IIb/IIIa and dual role of epinephrine', *Proc. Natl. Acad. Sci. USA* 1986, 83: 9197–9201.
5. Berndt, M. C. and Phillips, D. R., 'Purification and preliminary physico-chemical characterization of human platelet membrane glycoprotein V', *J. Biol. Chem.* 1981, 256: 59–65.
6. Berndt, M. C., Chong, B. H., Bull, H. A., Zola, Z., and Castaldi, P. A., 'Molecular characterization of quinine/quinidine drug dependent antibody platelet interaction using monoclonal antibodies', *Blood* 1985, 66: 1292–1301.
7. Bray, P. F., Rosa, J.-P., Lingappa, V. R., Kahn, Y. W., McEver, R. P., and Shuman, M. A., 'Biogenesis of the platelet receptor for fibrinogen: evidence for separate precursors for glycoprotein IIb and IIIa', *Proc. Natl. Acad. Sci. USA* 1986, 83: 1480–1484.
8. Calvete, J. J., Henschen, A., and Gonzalez-Rodriguez, J., 'Assignment of disulphide bonds in human platelet GPIIIa. A disulphide pattern for the β-subunits of the integrin family', *Biochem. J.* 1991, 274: 63–71.
9. Charo, I. F., Nannizzi, L., Phillips, D. R., Hsu, M. A., and Scarborrough, R. M., 'Inhibition of fibrinogen binding to GPIIb-IIIa by a GPIIIa peptide', *J. Biol. Chem.* 1991, 266: 1415–1421.
10. Cheresh, D. A., Berliner, S. A., Vincente, V., and Ruggeri, Z., 'Recognition of distinct adhesive sites on fibrinogen by related integrins on platelets and endothelial cells', *Cell* 1989, 58: 945–953.
11. Clemetson, K. J., 'Glycoproteins of the platelet plasma membrane', in: *Platelet Membrane Glycoproteins*, George, J. N., Nurden, A. T., Phillips, D. R. (Eds.), 1985, 51–85, Plenum Press, New York.
12. Deckmyn, H., van Houtte E., and Vermylen, J., 'Disturbed platelet aggregation to collagen associated with an antibody against an 85–90 Kd platelet glycoprotein in a patient with prolonged bleeding time', *Blood* 1992, 79: 1466–1471.
13. Doolittle, R. F., Watt, K. W. K., Cottrell, B. A., Strong, D. D., and Riley, M., 'The amino acid sequence of the a chain of human fibrinogen', *Nature* 1979, 280: 464–467.
14. D'Souza, S. E., Ginsberg, M. H., Burke, T. A., Lam, S. C.-T., and Plow, E. F., 'Localization of an Arg-Gly-Asp recognition site within an integrin receptor', *Science* 1988, 242: 91–93.
15. D'Souza, S. E., Ginsberg, M. H. Burke, T. A., and Plow, E. D., 'The ligand binding site of the platelet integrin receptor GPIIb-IIIa is proximal to the second calcium binding domain of its α subunit', *J. Biol. Chem.* 1990, 265: 3440–3446.
16. D'Souza, S. E., Ginsberg, M. H., Matsueda, G. R., and Plow, E. F., 'A discrete sequence in a platelet integrin is involved in ligand recognition', *Nature* 1991, 350: 66–68.
17. Du, X., Plow, E. F., Frelinger,III, A. L., O'Toole, T. E., Loftus, J. C., and Ginsberg, M. H., 'Ligands activate integrin $\alpha_{IIb}\beta_3$ (Platelet GPIIb-IIIa)', *Cell* 1991, 65: 409–416.
18. Du, X., Beutler, L., Ruan, C., Castaldi, P. A., and Berndt, M. C., 'Glycoprotein Ib and glycoprotein IX are fully complexed in the intact platelet membrane', *Blood* 1987, 69: 1524–1527.
19. Ezzell, R. M., Kenney, D. M., Egan, S., Stossel, T. P., and Hartwig, J. H., 'Localization of the domain of actin-binding protein that binds to membrane glycoprotein Ib and actin in human platelets', *J. Biol. Chem.* 1988, 263: 13303–13309.
20. Feizi, T., 'Carbohydrate differentiation antigens: probable ligands for cell adhesion molecules', *Trends in Biochem. Sci.* 1991, 16: 84–86.
21. Ferrell, J. E. and Martin, G. S., 'Tyrosine-specific protein phosphorylation is regulated by glycoprotein IIb-IIIa in platelets', *Proc. Natl. Acad. Sci. USA* 1989, 86: 2234–2238.
22. Fitzgerald, L. A., Steiner, B., Rall, S. C., Lo, S. S., and Phillips, D. R., 'Protein sequence

of endothelial cell glycoprotein IIIa derived from a cDNA clone. Identity with platelet GPIIIa and similarity with "integrin"', *J. Biol. Chem.* 1987, 262: 3936–3939.

23. Fox, J. E. B., Aggerbeck, L. A., and Berndt, M. C., 'Structure of the glycoprotein Ib-IX complex from platelet membranes', *J. Biol. Chem.* 1988, 263: 4882–4890.
24. Fox, J. E. B., Boyles, J. K., Berndt, M. C., Steffen, P. K,. and Anderson, L. K., 'Identification of a membrane skeleton in platelets', *J. Cell Biol.* 1988, 106: 1525–1538.
25. Fox, J. E. B., Reynolds, C. C., and Johnson, M. M., 'Identification Ibβ as one of the major proteins phosphorylated during exposure of intact platelets to agents that activate cyclic AMP-dependent protein kinase', *J. Biol. Chem.* 1987, 262: 12627–12631.
26. Frelinger, A. L., Lam, S. C.-T., Plow, E. F., Smith, M. A., Loftus, J. C., and Ginsberg, M. H., 'Occupancy of an adhesive glycoprotein receptor modulates expression of an antigenic site involved in cell adhesion', *J. Biol. Chem.* 1988, 263: 12397–12402.
27. Frelinger, A. L., Du, Xiaoping, Plow, E. F., and Ginsberg, M. H., 'Monoclonal antibodies to ligand-occupied conformers of integrin $\alpha_{IIb}\beta_3$ (glycoprotein GPIIb-IIIa) alter receptor affinity, specificity, and function', *J. Biol. Chem.* 1991, 266: 17106–17111.
28. Fujimura, Y., Titani, K., Holland, L. Z., Russell, S. R., Roberts, J. R., Elder, J. H., Ruggeri, Z. M., and Zimmerman, T. S., 'Von Willebrand factor. A reduced and alkylated 52/48-kDa fragment beginning at amino acid residue 449 contains the domain interacting with platelet glycoprotein Ib', *J. Biol. Chem.* 1986, 261: 381–385.
29. George, J. N., Nurden, A. T., and Phillips, D. R., 'Molecular defects in interactions of platelets with the vessel wall', *N. Engl. J. Med.* 1984, 311: 1084–1098.
30. George, J. N., Caen J. P., and Nurden, A. T., 'Glanzmann's thrombasthenia: the spectrum of clinical disease', *Blood* 1990, 75: 1383–1395.
31. Golden, A., Brugge, J. S., and Shattil, S., 'Role of platelet membrane glycoprotein IIb-IIIa in agonist-induced tyrosine phosphorylation of platelet proteins', *J. Cell. Biol.* 1990, 111: 3117–3127.
32. Gulino, D., Ryckewaert, J. J., Andrieux, A., Rabiet, M. J., and Marguerie, G., 'Identification of a monoclonal antibody against platelet GPIIb that interacts with a calcium binding site and induces aggregation', *J. Biol. Chem.* 1990, 265: 9575–9581.
33. Hamburger, S. A. and McEver, R. P., 'GMP–140 mediates adhesion of stimulated platelets to neutrophils', *Blood* 1990, 75: 550–554.
34. Harmon, J. T. and Jamieson, G. A., 'The glycocalacin portion of platelet glycoprotein Ib expresses both high and moderate affinity receptor sites for thrombin. A soluble radioreceptor assay for the interaction of thrombin with platelets', *J. Biol. Chem.* 1986, 261: 13224–13229.
35. Hickey, M. J., Williams, S. A., and Roth, G. J., 'Human platelet glycoprotein IX: an adhesive prototype of leucine-rich glycoproteins with flank-center-flank structures', *Proc. Natl. Acad. Sci. USA* 1989, 86: 6773–6777.
36. Hillery, C. A., Smyth, S. S., and Parise, L. V., 'Phosphorylation of human platelet glycoprotein IIIa (GPIIIa). Dissociation from fibrinogen receptor activation and phosphorylation of GPIIIa in vitro', *J. Biol. Chem.* 1991, 266: 14663–14669.
37. Huang, M., Bolen, J., Barnwell, J., and Shattil, S., 'Membrane glycoprotein IV (CD36) is physically associated with the Fyn, Lyn, and Yes protein-tyrosine kinases in human platelets', *Proc. Natl. Acad. Sci. USA* 1991, 88: 7844–7848.
38. Hynes, R. O., 'Integrins: a family of cell surface receptors', *Cell* 1987, 48: 549–554.
39. Hynes, R. O., 'The complexity of platelet adhesion to extracellular matrices', *Thrombosis and Haemostasis* 1991, 66: 40–43.
40. Hynes R. and Lander A., 'Contact and adhesive specificities in the associations, migrations, and targeting of cells and axons', *Cell* 1992, 68: 303–322.
41. Hynes R. O., 'Integrins: versatility, modulation, and signaling in cell adhesion', *Cell* 1992, 69: 11–25.
42. Isenberg, W. M., McEver, R. P., Phillips, D. R., Shuman, M. A., and Bainton, D. F., 'The platelet fibrinogen receptor: An immunogold-surface replica study of agonist-induced ligand binding and receptor clustering', *J. Cell. Biol.* 1987, 104: 1655–1663.

43. Johnston, G. I., Cook, R. G., and McEver, R. P., 'Cloning of GMP–140, a granule membrane protein of platelets and endothelium: Sequence similarity to proteins involved in cell adhesion and inflammation', *Cell* 1989, 56: 1033–1044.
44. Kieffer, N., Fitzgerald, L. A., Wolf, D. L., Cheresh, D. A., and Phillips, D. R., 'Adhesive properties of the $\beta 3$ integrins: Comparison of GPIIb-IIIa and the vitronectin receptor individually expressed in human melanoma cells', *J. Cell. Biol.* 1991, 113: 451–461.
45. Kieffer, N. and Matsueda, G., 'Resting GPIIb-IIIa interaction with immobilized fibrinogen is mediated through the fibrinogen γ chain dodecapeptide', *Blood* 1991, 78 (suppl.1) 1113 (Abtr.)
46. Kieffer N. and Phillips D., 'Platelet membrane glycoproteins: functions in cellular interactions', *Annu. Rev. Cell. Biol.* 1990, 6: 329–357.
47. Kieffer, N., Nurden, A. T., Hasitz, M., Titeux, M., and Breton-Gorius, J., 'Identification of platelet membrane thrombospondin binding molecules using an anti- thrombospondin antibody', *Biochim. Biophys. Acta* 1988, 967: 408–415.
48. Kloczewiak, M. Timmons, S., Bednarek, A., Sakon, M., and Hawiger, J., 'Platelet receptor recognition domain on the γ chain of human fibrinogen and its synthetic peptide analogues', *Biochemistry* 1989, 28: 2915–2919.
49. Knapp, W., Dörken, B., Rieber, P., Schmidt, R. E., Stein, H., and von dem Borne, A. E. G., 'CD Antigens 1989', *Blood* 1989, 74: 1448–1450.
50. Kouns, W. C., Wall, C. D., White, M. M., Fox, C. F., and Jennings, L., 'A conformation-dependent epitope of human platelet glycoprotein IIIa', *J. Biol. Chem.* 1990, 265: 20594–20601.
51. Lam, S. C., Plow, E., Smith, M. A., Andrieux, A., Ryckewaert, J., *et al.*, 'Evidence that the arginyl-glycyl-aspartate peptides and fibrinogen γ chain peptides share a common binding site on platelets', *J. Biol. Chem.* 1987, 262: 947–950.
52. Larsen, E., Celi, A., Gilbert, G. E., Furie, B. C., Erban, J. K., Bonfanti, R., Wagner, D. D., and Furie, B., 'PADGEM protein: A receptor that mediates the interaction of activated platelets with neutrophils and monocytes', *Cell* 1989, 59: 305–312.
53. Leung, L. L. K., 'Role of thrombospondin in platelet aggregation', *J. Clin. Invest.* 1984, 74: 1764–1772.
54. Leung, L. L. K., Li, W., McGregor, J. L., Albrecht, G., and Howard, R. J., 'CD36 synthetic peptides enhance or inhibit CD36-thrombospondin binding. A two step process of ligand-receptor interaction', *Blood* 1991, 78: (Suppl.1) 722 (Abstr.).
55. Loike, J. D., Sodeik, B., Cao, L., Leucona, S., Weitz, J., Detmers, P., Wright, S., and Silverstein, S., 'CD11c/CD18 on neutrophils recognizes a domain at the N terminus of the Aα chain of fibrinogen', *Proc. Natl. Acad. Sci. USA* 1991, 88: 1044–1048.
56. Lopez, J. A., Chung, D. W., Fujikawa, K., Hagen, F. S., Davie, E. W., and Roth, G. J., 'The α and β chains of human platelet glycoprotein Ib are both transmembrane proteins containing a leucine-rich amino acid sequence', *Proc. Natl. Acad. Sci. USA* 1988, 85: 2135–2139.
57. Lopez, J. A., Chung, D. W., Fujikawa, K., Hagen, F. S., Papayannopoulou, T., and Roth, G. J., 'Cloning of the α chain of human platelet glycoprotein Ib: a transmembrane protein with homology to leucine-rich α_2-glycoprotein', *Proc. Natl. Acad. Sci. USA* 1987, 84: 5615–5619.
58. Manning, D. and Brass, L., 'The role of GTP-binding proteins in platelet activation', *Thromb. Haemost.* 1991, 66: 393–399.
59. McEver, R. P., 'Leukocyte interactions mediated by selectins', *Thromb. Haemost.* 1991, 66: 80–87.
60. McGregor, J. L., Catimel, B., Parmentier, S., Clezardin, P., Dechavanne, M., and Leung, L. L. K., 'Rapid purification and partial characterization of human platelet glycoprotein IIIb', *J. Biol. Chem.* 1989, 264: 501–506.
61. Modderman, P. W., Admiraal, L. G., Sonnenberg, A., and Borne, A. E. G. K. V., 'Glycoprotein-V and glycoprotein-Ib-IX form a noncovalent complex in the platelet membrane', *Journal of Biological Chemistry* 1992, 267: 364–369.

62. Mohri, H., Yoshioka, A., Zimmerman, T. S., and Ruggeri, Z. M., 'Isolation of the von Willebrand factor domain interacting with platelet glycoprotein Ib, heparin, and collagen and characterization of its three distinct functional sites', *J. Biol. Chem.* 1989, 264: 17361–17367.
63. Moroi, M., Jung, S., Okuma M., and Shinmyozu K., 'A patient with platelets deficient in glycoprotein VI that lack both collagen-induced aggregation and adhesion', *J. Clin. Invest.* 1989, 84: 1440–1445.
64. Newman, P. J., Berndt, N. C., Gorski, J., White, G. C. II, Lyman, S., Paddock, C., and Muller, W. A., 'PECAM-1 (CD31) cloning and relation to adhesion molecules of the immunoglobulin gene super family', *Science* 1990, 247: 1219–1222.
65. Oquendo, P. Hundt, E., Lawler, J., and Seed, B., 'CD36 directly mediates cytoadherence of *Plasmodium falciparum* parasitized erythrocytes', *Cell* 1989, 58: 95–101.
66. O'Toole, T. E., Loftus, J. C., Plow, E. F., Glass, A. A., Harper, J. R., and Ginsberg, M., 'Efficient surface expression of platelet GPIIb-IIIa requires both subunits', *Blood* 1989, 74: 14–18.
67. O'Toole, T. E., Mandelman, D., Forsyth, J., Shattil, S., Plow, E. F., and Ginsberg, M. H., 'Modulation of the affinity of integrin $\alpha_{IIb}\beta_3$ (GPIIb-IIIa) by the cytoplasmic domain of αIIb', *Science* 1991, 254: 845–847.
68. Parise, L. V., Helgerson, S. L., Steiner, B., Nannizzi, L., and Phillips, D. R., 'Synthetic peptides derived from fibrinogen and fibronectin change the conformation of purified platelet glycoprotein IIb-IIIa', *J. Biol. Chem.* 1987, 262: 12597–12602.
69. Parise, L., Criss, A., Nannizzi, L., and Wardell, M. R., 'Glycoprotein IIIa is phosphorylated in intact platelets', *Blood* 1990, 75: 2363–2368.
70. Phillips, D., Charo, I., and Scarborrough R., 'GPIIb-IIIa: the responsive integrin', *Cell* 1991, 65: 359–362.
71. Phillips, D. R., Charo, I. F., Parise, L. V., and Fitzgerald, L. A., 'The platelet membrane glycoprotein IIb-IIIa complex', *Blood* 1988, 71: 831–843.
72. Pidard, D., Frelinger, A., Bouillot, C., and Nurden, A. T., 'Activation of the fibrinogen receptor on human platelets exposed to alpha-chymotrypsin – relationship with a major proteolytic cleavage at the carboxyterminus of the membrane glycoprotein-IIb heavy chain', *Eur. J. Biochem.* 1991, 200: 437–447.
73. Poncz, M., Eisman, R., Heidenreich, R., Silver, S. M., Vilaire, G., Surrey, S., Schwartz, E., and Bennett, J. S., 'Structure of the platelet membrane glycoprotein IIb: homology to the a subunits of the vitronectin and fibronectin membrane receptors', *J. Biol. Chem.* 1987, 262: 8476–8482.
74. Rosa, J. P., Bray, P., Gayet, O., Johnston, G., Cook, R., Jackson, K., Shuman, M., and McEver, R., 'Cloning of glycoprotein IIIa cDNA from human erythroleukemic cells and localization of the gene to chromosome 17', *Blood* 1988, 72: 593–600.
75. Roth, G. J., Church, T. A., McMullen, B. A., and Williams, S. A., 'Human platelet glycoprotein V: a surface leucine-rich glycoprotein related to adhesion', *Biochem. Biophys. Res. Commun.* 1990, 170: 153–161.
76. Roth, G. J., 'Developing relationships: Arterial platelet adhesion, glycoprotein Ib and leucine-rich glycoproteins', *Blood* 1991, 77: 5–19.
77. Savage, B. and Ruggeri, Z. M., 'Selective recognition of adhesive sites in surface-bound fibrinogen by glycoprotein IIb-IIIa on nonactivated platelets', *J. Biol. Chem.* 1991, 266: 11227–11233.
78. Schimomura, T., Fujimura, K., Maehama, S., Takemoto, M., Oda, K., Fujimoto, T., Oyama, R., Suzuki, M., Ichihara-Tanaka, K., Titani, K., and Kuramoto, A., 'Rapid purification and characterization of human platelet glycoprotein V: the amino acid sequence contains leucine-rich repetitive modules as in glycoprotein Ib', *Blood* 1990, 75: 2349–2356.
79. Sims, P. J., Ginsberg, M. H., Plow, E. F., and Shattil, S. J., 'Effect of platelet activation on the conformation of the plasma membrane glycoprotein IIb-IIIa complex', *J. Biol. Chem.* 1991, 266: 7345–7352.

80. Shattil, S. J., Hoxie, J., Cunningham, M., and Brass, L., 'Changes in the platelet membrane glycoprotein IIb-IIIa complex during platelet activation', *J. Biol. Chem.* 1985, 260: 11107–11114.
81. Sultan, C., Plantavid, M., Bachelot, C., Grondin, P., Breton, M., Mauco, G., Levy-Toledano, S., Caen, J. P., and Chap, H., 'Involvement of platelet glycoprotein IIb-IIIa (alphaIIb-beta3 Integrin) in thrombin-induced synthesis of phosphatidylinositol 3′,4′-bisphosphate', *J. Biol. Chem.* 1991, 266: 23554–23557.
82. Takahashi, N., Takahishi, Y., and Putman, F. W., 'Periodicity of leucine and tandem repetition of a 24 amino acid segment in the primary structure of leucine rich α_2-glycoprotein of human serum', *Proc. Natl. Acad. Sci. USA* 1985, 82: 1906–1910.
83. Tandon, N. N., Lipsky, R. H., Murgess, W. H., and Jamieson, G. A., 'Isolation and characterization of platelet glycoprotein IV (CD36)', *J. Biol. Chem.* 1989, 264: 7570–7575.
84. Tandon, N., Kralisc, U., and Jamieson, G. A., 'Identification of glycoprotein IV (CD36) as a primary receptor for platelet-collagen adhesion', *J. Biol. Chem.* 1989, 264: 7576–7583.
85. van Mourik, J. A., Leeksma, O. C., Reinders, J. H., Groot, P. G. de, and Zandbergen-Spaargaren, J., 'Vascular endothelial cells synthesize a plasma membrane protein indistinguishable from the platelet membrane glycoprotein IIa', *J. Biol. Chem.* 1985, 260: 11300–11306.
86. van Willigen, G. and Akkerman, J., 'Regulation of glycoprotein GPIIb-IIIa exposure on platelets stimulated with α-thrombin', *Blood* 1992, 79: 82–90.
87. van Willigen, G. and Akkerman, J., 'Protein kinase C and cyclic AMP regulate reversible exposure of binding sites for fibrinogen on the glycoprotein IIb-IIIa complex of human platelets', *Biochem. J.* 1991, 273: 115–120.
88. Vincente, V., Houghten, R. A., and Ruggeri, Z. M., 'Identification of a site in the α chain of platelet glycoprotein Ib that participates in von Willebrand factor binding', *J. Biol. Chem.* 1990, 265: 274–280.
89. Weiss, H. J., Turitto, V. T., and Baumgartner, H. R., 'Platelet adhesion and thrombus formation on subendothelium in platelets deficient in glycoproteins IIb-IIIa, Ib and storage granules', *Blood* 1986, 67: 322–330.
90. Wyler, B., Bienz, D., Clemetson, K. J., and Luscher, E. F., 'Glycoprotein Ibβ is the only phosphorylated major membrane glycoprotein in human platelets', *Biochem. J.* 1986, 234: 373–379.
91. Yamamoto, N., Ikeda, H., Tandon, N., Herman, J., Tomiyama, Y., Mitani, T., Sekuiguchi, S., Lipsky, R., Kralisz, U., and Jamieson G., 'A platelet membrane glycoprotein (GP) deficiency in healthy blood donors: Nak^{a-}-platelets lack detectable GPIV (CD36)', *Blood* 1990, 76: 1698–1703.
92. Zamarron, C., Ginsberg, M. H. and Plow, E. F., 'A receptor-induced binding site in fibrinogen elicited by its interaction with platelet membrane glycoprotein-IIb-IIIa', *J. Biol. Chem.* 1991, 266: 16193–16199.
93. Zehnder, J. L., Hirai, K., Shatsky, M., McGregor, J. L., Levitt, L. J., and Leung, L. L. K., 'The Cell Adhesion Molecule CD31 Is Phosphorylated After Cell Activation – Down-Regulation of CD31 in Activated Lymphocytes-T', *J. Biol. Chem.* 1992, 267: 5243–5249.

3. Platelet immunology: allo-antigens, transfusion

B. BOVAL, J. P. FEUGEAS and J.-L. WAUTIER
Hématologie – Transfusion, Hôpital Lariboisière, 2 Rue Ambroise Paré, 75010 Paris, France

Introduction

Platelet transfusions were introduced in the early sixties. However they have only been developed when plastic bags could be used as blood containers. Another important step was achieved when cell separators have permit to obtain large amount from one blood donor. Platelet transfusions are now a common therapeutical approach of primary thrombocytopenia or cytopenia secondary to chemotherapy. Their development has pointed out two aspects: first the role of platelet alloantigen, second the importance of the technique used to collect platelet and the conditions of platelet storage.

Human platelet antigens

In the last decade several platelet antigens were identified. The first diallelic system (PL^{A1} or Zw^{a}) was simultaneously described in the Netherlands and in USA; the report of cases of post transfusionnal purpura (PTP) or neo natal allo immune thrombocytopenia has permit to identify new antigen determinants, but the small amount of the serum samples, the high frequency of contaminating anti HLA antibodies were limitating factors for a good characterization of these antigens. The development of new techniques applied in platelet immunology such as flow cytometry, ELISA techniques, MAIPA techniques or Western blotting, has led to the discovery of a number of new platelet specific alloantigens. Then progress has been made by the use of new technologies: molecular biology, monoclonal antibodies. The need of a uniform nomenclature was achieved with the increase of specific platelet antigens. They are now named Human Platelet Antigen (HPA) [1].

HPA–1 system

This system was first described by Van Loghem [2] as Zw^{a} antigen and by Shulman [3] as Pl^{A1} antigen. Now named HPA–1 according to the new nomenclature, this system consists in two alloantigens: HPA–1a and HPA–1b with a respective genomic frequency of 85% and 15% in the Caucasian population, and a phenotypic frequency of 97.9% and 26.5%. These antigens have been defined by antibodies found in the sera of patients with post transfusionnal purpura. The PTP is a thrombocytopenic purpura occuring 6 to 14

Y. F. Missirlis and J.-L. Wautier (eds.), The Role of Platelets in Blood-Biomaterial Interactions, 33–44.

days after transfusion (packed red cells essentially). The highest number of the patients are female (in a series of 104 observations of PTP, 99 patients were women). All subjects have been preimmunized during a pregnancy and or by previous blood transfusion. Thrombocytopenia is often severe and the platelet count lower than 10^9 platelets /l in 81% of cases [4]. Some patients (5 to 10%) died from intracerebral haemorrhage. In most of the cases, the patients recovered a normal platelet count within two weeks. Different treatments have been proposed including corticotherapy, plasma exchange, intravenous immunoglobulins or compatible platelet transfusion. Some antibodies anti HPA–1 are responsible for allo immune neonatal thrombocytopenia: the maternal platelet specific antibodies crossing placental barrier, can induce fetal platelet destruction or at birth the baby may be thrombocytopenic. In fact, platelet antigens (especially HPA–1a) are expressed very early on fetal platelets [5]. A relationship between HLA haplotype HLA-B8,DR3 and alloimmunization anti HPA–1a is frequently observed [6]. HPA–1 antigens are located on platelet glycoprotein GP IIIa , absent in type I Glanzmann thrombasthenia [7]. Peptides study and nucleotide sequence coding for HPA–1 antigens demonstrated that the substitution in position 33 of a leucine by a proline aminoacid corresponds to a difference of the 196 base of DNA (C-T) [8].

HPA–2 system

The two antigens (HPA–2a, HPA–2b) of this platelet group were first reported in 1961, 1962 and named respectively Ko^b, Ko^a [9]. They were found in sera of multitransfused patients. Later anti Sib^a has been recognized as identical to anti Ko^a. HPA–2a is present in a large majority on platelets of Caucasian people (99.3%), and localized on N terminal globular fragment of platelet glycoprotein Ib alpha, absent in Bernard Soulier syndrome [10]. A substitution Threonine-Methionine in position 145 of the peptide of this part of the GP Ib is responsible for phenotypic expression [11].

HPA–3 system

The two antigens of this diallelic system were first reported in a case of faeto-maternal immunization and named Bak^a [12], and at the same time described in a case of PTP under Lek^a denomination [13]. The frequency of HPA–3a is slightly lower than the other antigens (87.7% phenotype frequency in Caucasian subjects). The antigens HPA–3a and HPA–3b are represented on platelet glycoprotein GP IIb, absent or at a low level in Glanzmann thrombasthenia [7]. Molecular basis of HPA–3 phenotype is a polymorphism in position 843, substitution of an isoleucine by a serine [14].

HPA–4 system

This system has been distinguished in 1985. The two antigens were named Pen^a (or Yuk^b) [15] and Pen^b (or Yuk^a) [16] . The anti HPA–4 antiplatelet antibodies were found during pregnancies leading to neonatal thrombocytopenia. Antigens are located on platelet GP IIIa , on a different site than HPA–1 antigens [17].

HPA–5 system

These antigens were recently discovered (1988, 1989) [18, 19]. Several names were first attributed to this system: Br, Zav, Hc; the two antigens are transmitted according to an autosomal codominant modality. Antibodies against HPA–5b antigen were found in sera of multitransfused patients, anti HPA–5a in sera of pregnant women; epitopes of HPA–5 antigens are present on platelet glycoprotein GP Ia [20]. A high frequency of HLA-DRw6 type were found in subjects developing anti HPA–5 antibodies [21]. This platelet antigen could be responsible of a large part of allo immune neonatal thrombocytopenia.

Other platelet antigens

At least five other platelet antigens were also reported in the literature, but they were not included in the international nomenclature. The Duzo system, the first platelet specific antigen reported in 1957 [22] has not been well characterized since the amount of antibody was limited. The PL^{E} system, described in 1963 is probably located on platelet GP Ib. Anti PL^{E1} antibody react with all tested platelets, but not with the platelets of the propositus. It seems that this patient suffered from a Bernard Soulier like syndrome [23]. Anti PL^{E2} serum is no longer available. Nak system has been reported in Japan and should be located on platelet glycoprotein GP IV [24]. It is involved in refractoriness to HLA matched platelet transfusions. A new system named Gov has two codominant alleles and is expressed on a platelet glycoprotein of 175 kd molecular weight [25]. One private platelet group have been described: platelet antigen Sr^{a}, located on platelet glycoprotein GP III.

Many of the platelet glycoproteins which carry platelet antigens belong to the adhesion molecules of the integrin superfamily . This explains why platelet antigens may be expressed not only on platelets but also on other cells (smooth muscle cells, endothelial cells, activated T cells). They are not platelet specific as it was thought previously. The role of carbohydrates on platelet glycoproteins is not well elucidated. Outside constitutional thrombopathies, no other association with diseases have been described. Phenotypic frequencies of these systems seem different according to ethnies, but no systematic anthropological studies have been conducted. In Table 1, we report phenotypic frequencies in Caucasian and Japanese populations of the five HPA systems.

Platelet collection

Therapeutic value of transfused platelets has been early demonstrated in this century. In the 1960s, platelet therapy was accomplished by transfusing whole blood, but storage conditions, adequate for whole blood were not acceptable

TABLE 1

Human platelet alloantigen systems: phenotype frequency (%) in Caucasian and Japanese populations.

System	Antigens	Other names	Phenotype frequency (%) Caucasian	Japanese
HPA-1	HPA-1a	Zw^a, Pl^{A1}	97.9	99.9
	HPA-1b	Zw^b, Pl^{A2}	26.5	3.7
HPA-2	HPA-2a	Ko^b	99.3	NT
	HPA-2b	Ko^a, Sib^a	14.6	25.4
HPA-3	HPA-3a	Bak^a, Lek^a	87.7	78.9
	HPA-3b	Bak^b	64.1	NT
HPA-4	HPA-4a	Pen^a, Yuk^b	99.9	99.9
	HPA-4b	Pen^b, Yuk^a	0.2	1.7
HPA-5	HPA-5a	Br^b, Zav^b	99.2	NT
	HPA-5b	Br^a, Zav^a, Hc^a	20.6	NT

for a good quality of platelets to be infused. The advent of plastic bags, closed systems, new techniques of separation or of collection opened a new area for platelet transfusions.

Donor selection

Plateletpheresis donor or whole blood donor must need the standard selection criteria. Aspirin intake diminish effectiveness of transfused platelets if single donor collection is done. A good quality of venipuncture with skin preparation, assuring sterile collection is needed, since platelet preparations are often stored at room temperature.

Platelet collection

Two types of collection are now used: whole blood collection or single donor plateletpheresis.

Whole blood donation: up to 7 ml per kg of body weight, in a time less than 10 minutes with CPD, CPD A1 or ACD anticoagulant is performed. Presumably an excessive time of blood collection induces activation or thrombin generation at the venipuncture site, and then promotes local platelet consumption. After a short time of storage at 20, 24°C, differential centrifugation is applied and a random platelet concentrate is obtained. Platelets are resuspensed in 50 to 70 ml of plasma, and stored on a variety of platelet agitator. Statistically, the platelet concentrate contains 5.5×10^{10} platelets per unit; commonly therapeutic dose of random platelets is 1 unit for 10 kg of body weight. The large number of different donors, raised the problem of potential viral transmission, and also of HLA contamination of platelet concentrate, and at last of platelet antigen alloimmunization.

The development of apheresis technology enables Blood Banks to produce platelet concentrates from single donor. Since the early 1970s, this technology has been used when patients developed refractoriness to platelet transfusions. Different types of collecting systems were used; first, open system, with a rotating seal in the procedure, and various connections,and later cell separator with single or dual stage channels (IBM 2997, COBE Laboratories, Lakewood, CO, USA). More recently apheresis has been performed with a totally closed system without rotating seal (CS–3000 cell separator, FENWAL Laboratories, Deerfield, IL, USA). The dual stage channel provide platelet concentrate of high purity, with extremely low contamination by red cells or white cells. A similar system, in total closed system have been developed using a SPECTRA separator (COBE Laboratories, USA). In a recent paper, Bertholf reported the performance of SPECTRA separator versus CS 3000 [28], during 31 procedures. Equivalent platelet yields were obtained with the two machines: 5.3×10^{11} platelets for CS 3000, 5.7×10^{11} platelets for SPECTRA. All products contain less than 1 ml of red cells. The mean white blood cells contamination is of 1×10^8 for CS 3000 but is extremely low with the COBE system: 0.03×10^8 by platelet concentrate. The good quality of these products may represent a crucial step in platelet transfusion procedure.

Platelet storage

The quality of platelet storage depends on several factors:

Platelet collection and general conditions of storage
Before storage itself, platelet collection may induce alterations of the stored platelet functions. Standardized conditions must be employed. Whole blood is collected into an anticoagulant with a pH around 7.0 which is suitable for platelets. Platelets stored at room temperature produce lactic acid through glycolysis and accumulate carbon dioxide from oxydative phosphorylation, both resulting in a decrease of PH during storage. If the pH drops below 6.0, there is an irreversible loss of viability and recovery [29]. A minimum plasma volume of 50 to 70 ml is recommended to buffer against pH decrease during storage [30].

Centrifugation techniques must provide maximum number of platelets and minimum white cell contamination. Slichter and Harker propose to use 1000 $\times$ g for 9 min to obtain PRP (platelet-rich plasma) and 3000 $\times$ g for 20 min to isolate platelets from PRP [31]. Platelets can also be prepared by a buffy-coat method. Fijnher *et al.* [32] showed that this method leads to less activated state platelets than those prepared by PRP method.

Leukocyte contamination is limited by filtration to prevent alloimmunization associated with multiple random donor platelet transfusions. Platelet concentrate can be UV-irradiated, using a single dose of ultraviolet light known to abrogate mixt lymphocyte reaction. Ultraviolet irradiation avoids alloimmunization and irradiated platelet concentrates retain satisfactory *in vitro* storage characteristics and *in vivo* survival [33].

Storage temperature influences post storage viability [29]: platelets stored at 4°C are enable to recover their discoid shape and have a reduced survival times after transfusion [34]. Storage temperature must be maintained below 20°C or 22°C [35].

During storage, gentle horizontal agitation improves recovery and survival [36]. Major forms of agitation are linear, flat-bed shaking, ferris wheel-type circular rotation and elliptical rotation. In non agitated platelet concentrates, anaerobic metabolism increases. Agitation seems to facilitate the diffusion of oxygen through the storage medium [37].

Plastic containers

The plastic containers have a great importance in platelet storage: they must provide maximum gas exchange across the bag in order to permit aerobic metabolism in stored platelet concentrates. If not, there is an increase production of lactic acid which causes a rapid decline in pH. Moreover, plasticizer leaching from the container into the concentrates must be as low as possible. Finally platelet adhesion and activation onto the biomaterial has to be reduced.

The major advance in improving stored platelets has been provided by the use of oxygen through gas-permeable storage bags. The first containers were made of PVC (polyvinyl chloride) plasticized with the chemical DEHP (di 2-ethylhexyl phtalate) plasticizer and allowed 3 days of storage [29]. Then TEHTM (tri- 2-ethylhexyl trimellitate) plasticizer was used to improve the PVC bags. The oxygen and carbon dioxide transmission rates for these bags are 2 times greater than for DEHP-PVC [36]. In addition a 30 fold reduction in plasticizer accumulating in the platelet concentrates has been observed [38]. Those TEHTM-PVC bags allow for at least 5 days of storage. Second generation containers are now available which are more gas-permeable by decreasing the thickness of the plastic or increasing the size of the bags. They allow 7 days storage [39]. Due to possible bacterial contamination in the storage container, however, the recommended storage time is still 5 days [40]. Other containers are made of polyolefin formulated without liquid plasticizer and are the most permeable of available bags to oxygen and carbon dioxyde. They appear comparable with second generation PVC containers but should be used for higher concentration of platelets or when leukocyte concentration is high [38].

Platelet adhesion and activation in containers probably contribute to shorten platelet survival after transfusion [41]. Platelet adhesion onto biomaterials is a criteria of biocompatibility and is extensively studied for vascular grafts and extracorporeal circulations as cardiopulmonary by-pass and hemodialysis. Several techniques have been devised to assess platelet deposition *in vitro*. The two principal methods used currently are the morphometric and isotopic techniques. Morphogenesis of platelet adhered on the surface of biomaterials has been divided into five types in scanning electron microscope (SEM) [42] and permit to evaluate semiquantitatively platelet adhesion. Application of this method is limited by visual field of SEM. Isotopic techniques using ^{51}Cr-labelled or ^{111}In-labelled platelets enable simple and rapid measurement of platelets adhered on the surface of biomaterials [43, 44]. However, single adherent platelet cannot be distinguished from platelet aggregates or thrombi and platelet functions may be perturbed by the labelling process. Surface phase immunoassay using a monoclonal antibody directed specifically against platelet glycoprotein GP IIIa are actually developed [45]. Mechanisms of platelet adhesion involve at least two steps: protein adsorption and then cellular interactions with the protein-coated biomedical polymer surface leading to adhesion and activation of cells [46]. After adhesion of the initial monolayer of platelets (primary platelets), Sheppeck et coll [47] showed a requirement of GP Ib in the adhesion of secondary platelets on biomaterials. So platelet activation in bags is also controlled by composition of media in which platelets are resuspensed, plasma or synthetic media.

Plasma and synthetic media

The preservative solutions currently used for platelet storage in plasma are red blood cells preservatives. An ideal preservative for platelets does not actually exist. Storage in plasma with citrate does not prevent activation of the fibrinolytic and kallicrein systems. Platelet can be actived by thrombin generation. Platelet activation provides release of platelet granule contents and leads to the formation of thromboxane A2 [48], with alterations of platelet membrane glycoproteins GP Ib/IX and GP IIb/IIIa [49]. Some additives as prostaglandins or thrombin inhibitors may decrease platelet activation during storage [50]. Platelet adhesion and aggregation are reduced after 24 hr of storage with aprotinin. However aprotinin prevents neither the GP Ib alpha reduction nor the modifications of the functions of human platelets stored in their autologous plasma [50]. Finally, improvement of *in vivo* platelet function with any additive has not been demonstrated [40].

As demonstrated by several authors, synthetic media could be used instead of plasma for platelet storage. Holme *et al.* [51] have shown significant improvement of both *in vitro* and *in vivo* viability of platelets with a physiologic salt solution supplemented with glucose, bicarbonate and citrate. Murphy and coworkers [52] have demonstrated the importance of buffering capacity of bicarbonate.

Evaluation of stored platelet viability and function

In vivo and *in vitro* tests have been developed to appreciate viability and function of platelet concentrates in order to determine the best conditions of storage.

In vivo tests provide a direct evaluation of the efficiency of transfusion. A global evaluation is made by measuring the increase in platelet count after transfusion in thrombocytopenic patients. Schiffer *et al.* [53] standardize the measured increments one hour after the transfusion with Corrected Count Increment (CCI):

$$\frac{\text{absolute increment} \times \text{body surface area}(\text{m}^2)}{\text{number of platelets}(\times 10^{11})}.$$

Moreover, parameters as recovery and survival can be determined by transfusion of radiolabeled platelets in normal volunteers. The platelets are labeled with ^{51}Cr or ^{111}In and reinfused into the original donor [54]. Percentage of recovery and survival time of fresh unstored labeled autologous platelets are respectively 56% and 5.3 days [31]. Recovery and survival times of transfused platelets may be compared with those ideal values.

In vivo function of transfused platelets can be poorly evaluated by adhesion tests and bleeding time. For instance, Borchgrevink [55] measured *in vivo* adhesiveness by simultaneous counting platelets in capillaries (from a wound) and in venous blood. Normally, the number of platelets is reduced by 30% in the capillaries. Recently, Owens *et al.* developed *ex vivo* studies [56]. They labeled fresh and stored platelets from the same donors with ^{111}In or ^{51}Cr respectively. Then they simultaneously infused mixed labeled platelets. So they could study recovery and survival times of fresh and stored platelets and determined *ex vivo* functional behaviour of labeled platelets. They showed that platelets stored for 5 days recovered (*in vivo*) adhesion and aggregability capacities similar to that of fresh platelets.

In vitro tests used to evaluate platelet functions are not always correlated with hemostatic functions after transfusion. Platelet morphology is assessed by phase contrast or electron microscopy. Normal circulating platelets are disk-shaped cells. Other shapes (spheres, dendritic forms, balloons) correspond with an alteration of viability [57]; an optical apparatus has been developed by Bellhouse *et al.* [58], which correlates percentage of disks and light transmission at two stirring speeds. This system provides semiquantitative information on the number of discoid platelets.

Measurement of oxygen and carbon dioxyde tension and determination of lactate may complete pH measurement to evaluate the ability of stored platelets to maintain aerobic versus anaerobic metabolism.

The simple technique of hypotonic stress has been largely used. After an addition of an hypotonic solution, a spectrophotometer analysis shows a rapid drop in light absorption which corresponds with osmotic shock. Then a progressive return to the original level corresponds to a morphological modification and is related to *in vivo* recovery. However it does not correlate with hemostatic effectiveness [61].

Platelet activation can be indirectly determined by studying expression of glycoproteins released from alpha granules during platelet activation. For instance alpha granule membrane protein GMP 140 expression increases with time of storage and can be considered as a marker of activation [41]. Similary, platelet concentrates plasma levels of platelet factor 4 (PF4) correlates with platelet activation: a low concentration of PF4 in plasma is an indicator of intact alpha granules in non activated platelets [37].

Transfusion effectiveness can be appreciated by means of an *in vitro* perfusion technique as described by Mazzara *et al.* [62]. Denuded rabbit arterial segments mounted in annular chambers are exposed to blood drawn directly from the antecubital vein. This perfusion system allows the direct visualization of platelet-subendothelium interactions.

Conclusion

The major advance in improving platelet storage was the introduction of gas-permeable storage bags (second generation containers). Other improvements are less subtantial. Synthetic media might, however, provide better conditions of storage and could enhance safety of platelet transfusions. A great variety of *in vivo* and *in vitro* tests are now available to determine platelet viability and function. Both types of tests may assess the positive contributions of any new storage technique. If *in vivo* and *in vitro* tests well correlate and suggest a positive effect of a new method, it must be verified that this improvement is effectively associated with a clinical benefit.

References

1. von dem Borne, A.E.G.Kr. and Decary, F., 'ICSH/ISBT Working party on platelet serology', *Vox. Sang.* 1990, 58: 176.
2. van Loghem, J.J., Dorfmeyer, H. and van den Hart, M., 'Serological and genetical studies on a platelet antigen (Zw)', *Vox Sang.* 1959, 4: 161–169.
3. Shulman, N.R., Aster, R.H., Leitner A. and Hiller, M., 'Immuno-reaction involving platelets. V: post transfusion purpura due to a complement fixing antibody against a genetically controlled platelet antigen. A proposed mechanism for thrombocytopenia and its relevance in "autoimmunity"', *J. Clin. Invest.* 1961, 40: 1597–1620.
4. Mueller-Eckhardt, C., Kroll, H., Kiefel, V. and the members of the european PTP group, 'Post transfusion purpura', in: *Platelet Immunology: Fundamental and Clinical Aspects* 1990, Edited by Editions Inserm, John Lilley Eurotext; Paris, Londres; 206: 249–255.
5. Gruel, Y., Boizard, B., Daffos, F., Forestier, F., Caen, J. and Wautier, J.L., 'Determination of platelet antigens and glycoproteins in the human fetus', *Blood* 1986, 68: 488–492.
6. Reznikoff-Etievant, M.F., Muller, J.Y., Julien, F. and Patereau, C., 'An immune response gene linked to MHC in man', *Tissue Antigens* 1983, 22: 312–314.
7. Kieffer, N., Boizard, B., Didry, D., Wautier, J.L. and Nurden, A.T., 'Immunochemical characterization of the platelet specific alloantigen Lek^{a}. A comparison study with the Pl^{A1} alloantigen', *Blood* 1984, 64: 1212–1219.
8. Newman, P.J., Derbes, R.S. and Aster, R.H., 'The human platelet alloantigens, PL^{A1} and PL^{A2}, are associated with a leucine 33/ proline 33 aminoacid polymorphism in

membrane glycoprotein IIIa, and are distinguishable by DNA typing', *J. Clin. Invest.* 1989, 83: 1778–1781.

9. van der Weerdt, C.M., van de Wiel-Dorfmeyer, H., Engelfriet, C.P. and van Loghem, J.J., 'A new platelet antigen', *Proc. 8th Congr. Europ. Soc. Haemat. Wien* 1961, 379, Karger, Basel.
10. Kuijpers, R.W.A.M., Ouwehand, W.H., Bleeker, P.M.M., Christie, D. and von dem Borne A.E.G.Kr., 'Localization of the platelet-specific HPA–2 (Ko) alloantigens on the N-terminal globular fragment of platelet glycoprotein Ib alpha', *Blood* 1992, 79: 283–288.
11. Kuijpers, R.W.A.M., Faber, N.M., Cuypers, H.TH., Ouwehand, W.H. and von dem Borne, A.E.G.Kr., 'NH2-terminal globular domain of human platelet glycoprotein Ib alpha has a methionine 145/threonine 145 amino acid polymorphism, which is associated with the HPA–2 (Ko) alloantigens', *J. Clin. Invest.* 1992, 89: 381–384.
12. von dem Borne, A.E.K.Kr., von Riesz, E., Vergheught, F.W.A., ten Cate, J.W., Koppe, J.G., Engelfriet, C.P. and Nijenhuis, L.E., 'Bak^a, a new platelet-specific antigen involved in neonatal allo-immune thrombocytopenia', *Vox Sang.* 1980, 39: 113–120.
13. Boizard, B. and Wautier, J.L., 'Lek^a, a new platelet antigen absent in glanzmann thrombasthenia', *Vox. Sang.* 1984, 46: 47–54.
14. Lyman, S., Aster, R.H., Visentin, G.P. and Newman P.J., 'Polymorphism of human platelet membrane glycoprotein IIb associated with the BaK^a/BaK^b alloantigen system', *Blood* 1990, 75: 2343–2348.
15. Friedman, J.M. and Aster, R.H., Neonatal alloimune thrombocytopenic purpura and congenital porencelophaly in two siblings associated with a "new" maternal antiplatelet antibody', *Blood* 1985, 65: 1412–1415.
16. Shibata, Y., Miyayi, Y., Ichikawa, Y. and Matsuda, I., 'A new platelet antigen system, Yuk^a/Yuk^b', *Vox Sang.* 1986, 51: 334–336.
17. Furihata, K., Nugent, D.J., Bissonette, A. and Aster, R.H., 'On the association of the platelet specific alloantigen Pen^a with glycoprotein IIIa. Evidence for heterogeneity of glycoprotein IIIa', *J. Clin. Invest.* 1987, 80: 1624–1630.
18. Kiefel, V., Santoso, S., Katzmann, B. and Mueller-Eckhardt C., 'A new platelet specific alloantigen Br^a. Report of 4 cases with neonatal alloimune thrombocytopenia', *Vox Sang.* 1988, 54: 101–106.
19. Woods, V.L., Pischel, K.D., Avery, E.D. and Bluestein, M.G., 'Antigenic polymorphism of human very late activation protein–2 (platelet glycoprotein Ia-IIa). Platelet alloantigen Hc^a', *J. Clin. Invest.* 1989, 83: 978–985.
20. Santoso, S., Kiefel, V., Kroll, H. and Mueller-Eckardt, C., 'Immunochemical characterization of the new platelet alloantigen system Br^a/Br^b', *Br. J. Haematol.* 1989, 72: 191–198.
21. Mueller-Eckhardt, C., Kiefel, V., Kroll, H., Mueller-Eckhardt, G., 'HLA-DRw6, a new immune response marker for inmmunization against the platelet alloantigen Br^a', *Vox Sang.* 1989, 57: 90–91.
22. Moulinier, J., 'Iso-immunisation maternelle anti plaquettaire et purpura neo natal. Le systeme de groupe plaquettaire "DUZO"', *Proc. 6th Cong. Europ. Soc. Haematol. Copenhagen* 1957, 236: 817–820, Karger, Basel.
23. Furihata, K., Hunter, J., Aster, R.H., Koewing, G.R., Shulman, N.R. and Kunicki, T.J., 'Human anti Pl^{E1} antibody recognizes epitopes associated with the alpha subunit of platelet glyprotein Ib', *Br. J. Haematol.* 1988, 68: 103–110.
24. Tomiyama, Y., Take, H., Ikeda H., *et al.*, 'Identification of the platelet-specific alloantigen, Nak^a, on platelet membrane glycoprotein IV', *Blood* 1990, 75: 684–687.
25. Kelton, J.G., Smith, J.W., Horsewood, P., Humbert, J.R., Hayward, C.P.M. and Warkentin, T.E.: Gov^a/Gov^b alloantigen system on human platelets. Blood, 1990; 75, 2172–2176.
26. Kroll, H., Kiefel, V., Santoso, S. and Mueller-Eckhardt, C., 'Sr^a, a private platelet antigen on glycoprotein IIIa associated with neonatal alloimmune thrombocytopenia', *Blood* 1990, 76: 2296–2302.
27. von dem Borne, A.E.G.Kr. and Kuipjers, R.W.A.M., 'Platelet antigens, new aspects',

in: *Platelet Immunology: Fundamental and Clinical Aspects.* Colloque Inserm / John Libbey Eurotext. 1991, 206: 219–240.
28. Bertholf, M.F. and Mintz, P.D., 'Comparison of plateletpheresis using two cell separators and identical donors', *Transfusion* 1989, 29: 521–523.
29. Murphy, S., Sayar, S.N. and Gardner, F.H., 'Storage of platelet concentrates at 22 degrees C', *Blood* 1970, 35: 547–549.
30. Slichter, S.J., 'Optimum platelet concentrate preparation and storage', in: *Current Concepts in Tranfusion Therapy.* Arlington, VA: American Association of Blood banks. 1985, 1–26.
31. Slichter, S.J. and Harker, L.A., 'Preparation and storage of platelet concentrates', *Br. J. Haematol.* 1976, 34: 395–402.
32. Fijnheer, R., Piertersz, R.N.I., de Korte, D., Gouwerok, C.W., Dekker, W.J., Reesink, H.W. and Roos, D., 'Platelet activation during preparation of platelet concentrates: a comparison of the platelet-rich plasma and the buffy coat methods', *Transfusion* 1990, 30: 634–638.
33. Pamphilon, D.H., Potter, M., Cutts, M., Meenaghan, M., Rogers, W., Slade, R.R., Saunders, J., Tandy, N.P. and Fraser, I.D.,' Platelet concentrates irradiated with ultraviolet light retain satisfactory in vitro storage characteristics and in vivo survival', *Br. J. Haematol.* 1990, 75: 240–244.
34. Sturk, A., Burt, L.M., Hakvoort, T., ten Cate, J.W. and Crawford, N., 'The effect of storage on platelet morphology', *Transfusion* 1882, 22: 115–120.
35. Gottschall, J.L., Rzad L. and Aster, R.H., 'Studies of the minimum temperature at which human platelets can be stored with full maintenance of viability', *Transfusion* 1986, 26: 460–462.
36. Simon, T.L., Nelson, E.J., Carmen, R. and Murphy, S., 'Extension of platelet concentrate storage', *Transfusion* 1983, 23: 207–212.
37. Wallvik, J., Stenke, L. and Akerblom, O., 'The effect of different agitation modes on platelet metabolism, thromboxane formation, and alpha granular release during platelet storage', *Transfusion* 1990, 30: 639–643.
38. Grode, G., Miripol, J., Gerber J. and Buchholz, D.H., 'Extensed storage of platelets in a new plastic container', *Transfusion* 1985, 25: 204–208.
39. Hogge, D.E., Thompson, B.W. and Schiffer, C.A., 'Platelet storage for 7 days in second generation blood bags', *Transfusion* 1986, 26: 131–135.
40. Stack, G. and Snyder, E.L., 'Storage of platelet concentrate', in: *Blood Separaration and Plasma Fractionnation* 1991, 99–125, Wiley-Liss Inc.
41. Rinder, H.M., Murphy, M., Mitchell, J.G., Stocks, J., Ault, K.A. and Hillman, R.S., 'Progressive platelet activation with storage: evidence for shortened survival of activated platelets after transfusion', *Transfusion* 1991, 31: 409–414.
42. Xi, T.F., Wang, C.R., Lei, X.H. and Tian, W.H., 'Deformation and classification of the adhesive platelets on the surface of biomaterials', *Transactions of 3rd World Biomaterials Congress* 1988, 315–316.
43. Bowry, S.K., Courtney, J., Prentice, C.R. and Douglas, J.T., 'Utilisation of the platelet release reaction in the blood compatibility assessment of polymers', *Biomaterials* 1984, 5: 289–292.
44. Cazenave, J.P., Blondowska, D., Richardson, M., Kinlough-Rathbone, R., Packam, M.A. and Mustard, J.F., 'Quantitative radioisotopic measurement and scanning electron microscopic study of platelet adherence to collagen-coated surface and to subendothelium with a rotating probe device', *J. Lab. Clin. Med.* 1979, 93: 60–70.
45. Xi, T.F., Zhang, J.C., Tian, W.H., Wang, C.R., Lei, X.H., Wai, H.Y. and Ruan, C.G., 'New method to quantitate platelets adhered on biomaterials using monoclonal antibodies to human platelet membrane glycoprotein SZ 21', *Biomater. Artif. Cells Artif. Organs* 1990, 18: 423–435.
46. Anderson, J.M., Bonfield, T.L., Ziats, N.P., 'Protein adsorption and cellular adhesion and activation on biomedical polymers', *Int. Artif. Organs* 1990, 13: 375–382.

47. Sheppeck, R.A., Garrett, K.O., Bentz, M.L. and Johnson, P.C., 'Platelet adhesion on polyethylene', *ASAIO Transactions* 1991, 37: M260–M261.
48. Bode, A.P. and Miller, D.T., 'Generation and degradation of fibrinopeptde A in stored platelet concentrates', *Vox Sang.* 1986, 51: 192–196.
49. Michaelson, A.D. and Barnard M.R., 'Thrombin induced changes in platelet membrane glycoproteins Ib-Ic and IIb-IIIa', *Blood* 1987, 70: 1673–1678.
50. Mazoyer, E., Boizard-Boval, B., Pidard, D., Caen, J. and Wautier, J.L., 'Platelet membrane glycoproteins and platelet functions during storage in the presence of a proteinase inhibitor', *Thrombosis Res.* 1991, 62: 165–175.
51. Holme, S., Heaton, W.A. and Courtright, M., 'Improve in vivo and in vitro viability of platelet concentrates stored for seven days in a platelet additive solution', *Br. J. Haematol.* 1987, 66: 233–238.
52. Murphy, S., Kagen, L. and Holme, S., 'Platelet storage in synthetic media lacking glucose and bicarbonate', *Transfusion* 1991, 31: 16–20.
53. Schiffer, C.A., Lee, E.J., Ness, P.M. and Reilly, J., 'Clinical evaluation of platelet concentrates stored for one to five days', *Blood* 1986, 67: 1591–1594.
54. Heaton, W.A.L., '^{111}In and ^{51}Cr labelling of platelets. Are they comparable?', *Transfusion* 1986, 26: 157–164.
55. Borchgrevinck, C.F., 'A method for measuring platelet adhesiveness in vivo', *Acta Med. Scand.* 1960, 168: 157–164.
56. Owens, M., Holme, S., Heaton A., Sawyer S. and Cardinali, S., 'Post transfusion recovery of function of 5-day stored platelet concentrates', *Br. J. Haematol.* 1992, 80: 539–544.
57. Becker, G.A., Tuccelli, M., Kunicki T.J., Chalos, M.K. and Aster, R.H., 'Studies of platelet concentrates stored at 22 degrees C and 4 degrees C', *Transfusion* 1975, 13: 61–65.
58. Bellhouse, M.A., Ross, I., Entwistle, C.C. and Bellhouse, B.J., 'Optical measurement of the viability of stored human platelets', *Optics Laser Technol.* 1985, 17: 27–30.
59. Bellhouse, E.L., Inskip, M.J., Davis, J.G. and Entwistle, C.C., 'Pre-transfusion non invasive quality assessement of stored platelet concentrates', *Br. J. Haematol.* 1987, 66: 503–508.
60. Lee, V.S., Tarassenko, L. and Bellhouse, B.J., 'Platelet transfusion therapy: platelet concentrate preparation and storage', *J. Lab. Clin. Med.* 1980, 111: 371–383.
61. Valerie, C.R., Feingold, H. and Marchioni, L.D., 'The relation between response to hypotonic stress and the ^{51}Cr recovery in vivo of preserved platelets', *Transfusion* 1974, 14: 331–335.
62. Mazzara, R., Escolar, G., Garrido, M., Pereira, A., Castillo, R. and Ordinas, A., 'Evaluation of the transfusion effectiveness of various platelet concentrates by means of an vitro perfusion technique', *Transfusion* 1991, 31: 308–312.

4. Pharmacology of platelets

The role of platelets in blood-biomaterial interactions

J. A. DAVIES

Academic Unit of Medicine, Martin Wing, The General Infirmary, Leeds, UK

Introduction

When circulating blood comes in contact with an artificial surface, certain plasma proteins are deposited virtually instantaneously. Blood platelets, accordingly, do not make direct contact with artificial materials in the bloodstream, but interact with the surface layer of protein (Table 1). The nature of the surface-bound protein layer varies with the nature of the artificial surface and the way in which it is introduced in the circulation. However, most synthetic materials become coated predominantly with fibrinogen [1] which gradually changes with time so that eventually the surface does not react with anti-fibrinogen antibodies. Blood-surface interaction rapidly generates thrombin, through contact activation of the coagulation mechanism, and exposure of platelets to thrombin is likely to be a major pathway of platelet activation. Finally, exposure of blood to artificial surfaces may generate shear stresses, leading to mechanical activation of platelets.

Whatever the initial stimulus (or combination of stimuli) exposure of platelets in flowing blood to an artificial surface will generate the full response of shape-change, adhesion, the release reaction and aggregation. Under these conditions, the objective of diminishing platelet interactions with artificial surfaces can be approached either by inhibiting adhesion, or by interfering with subsequent platelet-platelet interaction and platelet aggregate formation (Table 2). Therapeutic applications have concentrated, at least until recently, on the latter approach because of the lack of agents which inhibited the initial phase of platelet adhesion. Moreover, in practical terms, adherence of a platelet monolayer on an exposed surface is unlikely to be deleterious in itself, but only in as far as it stimulates adhesion-induced aggregation.

Attempts to inhibit platelet activation at artificial surfaces have, in consequence, centred on the use of agents which inhibit pathways of platelet activation and which are not adhesion-specific.

Y. F. Missirlis and J.-L. Wautier (eds.), The Role of Platelets in Blood-Biomaterial Interactions, 45–57.

TABLE 1
Mechanisms of platelet activation at artificial surfaces.

• adhesion to adsorbed plasma proteins (fibrinogen, vWF, fibronectin, coagulation factors)
• generation of thrombin
• exposure to shear stress
• stimulation by release products of activated placelets

TABLE 2
Inhibition of platelet activation at artificial surfaces.

• interference with eicosanoid synthesis and metabolism
• inhibition of thrombin
• inhibition of adhesin binding
• other mechanisms

Interference with eicosanoid synthesis and metabolism

Generation of thrombin following blood-surface interaction is probably a key event in platelet activation by surfaces. Thrombin is a potent inducer of thromboxane A_2 synthesis by platelets [2]. Thrombin triggers release of arachidonate from the platelet membrane through the action of phospholipase A_2 and subsequent metabolism of arachidonate generates prostaglandin G_2 (PGG_2) PGH_2 and thromboxane A_2 (TXA_2) all potent pro-aggregatory compounds acting through the thromboxane receptor. Recognition of the importance of this pathway in platelet activation has been the impetus behind the synthesis and development of agents which block the thromboxane receptor or inhibit thromboxane synthesis.

Eicosanoid metabolism in endothelial (and other) cells in contrast leads to synthesis of prostaglandins D_2, E_2 and I_2 with opposing actions, inhibiting platelet adhesion, shape change and aggregation by activating adenylate cyclase [3] and raising platelet cyclic AMP. Recognition of the inhibitory potency particularly of PGI_2 has led to a therapeutic search for stable analogues, though clinical use has been hampered by its profound hypotensive effects.

Aspirin

Aspirin was effectively the first platelet inhibitor to be accepted in clinical practice and the fact that it is still by far the most widely used illustrates the difficulty of developing platelet inhibitor compounds. It acts by acetylating a hydroxyl group in the active centre of the enzyme cyclooxygenase [4] thereby inhibiting platelet synthesis of thromboxane and the unstable intermediates for the lifetime of the platelet. This action inhibits the second-phase of platelet aggregation induced by soluble agonists [5] though inhibition can be overcome by increasing the concentration of collagen or thrombin. Aspirin does not affect platelet adhesion and so does not prevent formation of the initial, surface-induced platelet monolayer [6].

Because it inhibits cyclooxygenase, aspirin similarly inhibits eicosanoid synthesis in vascular cells, blocking synthesis of PGI_2 [7]. On theoretical grounds this was held to have the potential risk of induction of platelet mediated thrombosis through suppression of PGI_2 production. This concern led to a proliferation of studies to find a dose of aspirin which preserved capacity for *in vivo* PGI_2 synthesis while inhibiting platelet function [8]. A level of less than 40 mg aspirin daily probably partly achieves this aim [9] but there is little evidence that in clinical practice this refinement is necessary and doses of aspirin which block PGI_2 production do not seem, in fact, to be pro-thrombotic.

Aspirin is a relatively weak platelet inhibitor, as might be predicted from its mechanism of action. Inhibition of cyclooxygenase does not block the main pathways of receptor-mediated platelet stimulation, so that platelet activation still occurs in response, for example, to thrombin or higher concentrations of ADP or collagen. This relative lack of efficacy can be illustrated by the effect on bleeding time in man, with prolongation by only 90 percent at steady-state levels following oral doses of 300 mg per day [10]. Nonetheless, numerous clinical studies have shown that aspirin is an effective anti-thrombotic agent, reducing vascular events in patients following treatment for myocardial infarction or stroke by 20–25 percent [11]. The discrepancy between its weak pharmacological action *in vitro* and the outcome of clinical studies lead to the suggestion that aspirin might have more general actions on haemostatic mechanisms, for example by impairment of coagulation protein synthesis, but evidence for this is lacking [10].

Aspirin does not inhibit shape change and platelet adhesion [6] though in experimental arterial injury it is effective in inhibiting platelet deposition on injured vascular surfaces [12]. Early reports of its efficacy in inhibiting platelet uptake on dialyser membranes depended on inhibition of secondary platelet-platelet interaction [13]. Aspirin may have a role as a supplementary therapy in prevention of thromboembolism in patients with mechanical heart-value prostheses who are already treated with warfarin, but carries a significant risk of excess bleeding [14].

Thromboxane synthesis inhibitors and thromboxane receptor blocking agents

These agents were developed at a time when there was concern that aspirin treatment had the adverse action of blocking synthesis of platelet inhibitor and vasodilator prostaglandins. Availability or otherwise of PGI_2 is not a major issue in the efficacy of platelet inhibitors at an artificial surface and so these agents might be expected to have a limited advantage over aspirin in suppression of platelet-surface interaction.

The rationale for development of thromboxane synthetase inhibitors was that by inhibiting thromboxane A_2 synthesis in platelets, the unstable metabolic precursors might be utilised for synthesis of PGI_2 in vascular cells, and PGD_2 in white-blood cells, thereby enhancing the platelet-inhibitory action. There was some evidence that this occurred on a small-scale when assessed *in vitro* [15]. However it became apparent that PGG_2 and PGH_2 could stimulate the thromboxane receptor so that anything less than 100 percent inhibition of thromboxane synthesis was liable to be ineffective. Thromboxane receptor antagonists avoid this disadvantage, preventing platelet stimulation by released, or exogenous thromboxane A_2 (as well as by PGG_2 and PGH_2). They maintain the (theoretical) advantage that synthesis of anti-aggregatory eicosanoids in other cells is not inhibited, though that apart, they should not exhibit other advantages over aspirin. Compounds combining thromboxane synthetase inhibitor activity and receptor blocking properties in one molecule have also been synthesised [16]. As might be predicted, these compounds inhibit platelet aggregation induced by low concentrations of ADP and collagen, and by high concentrations of arachidonate and thromboxane mimetic [17]. In whole blood, small increases in levels of PGD_2, PGE_2 and 6-keto-$PGF_{1\alpha}$ can be detected [18]. Whether because of this property, or some other mechanism, bleeding time following administration to volunteers was increased by a mean of 85% compared with a 25% increase following aspirin 1g in one study [17].

There has been limited clinical experience with these agents in the inhibition of platelet deposition on artificial surfaces. The thromboxane synthetase inhibitor, dazoxiban, was shown to reduce serum thromboxane B_2 levels in patients undergoing haemodyalisis, but did not reduce platelet loss in the dialyser, nor reduce the requirement for heparin [18]. The thromboxane receptor blocking agent AH23848 in contrast inhibited platelet deposition on aorto-bifemoral Dacron grafts in man and was significantly more effective than a combination of aspirin and dipyridamole [19].

Prostaglandin I_2

Prostaglandin I_2 was first described in 1978 as an eicosanoid synthesized by endothelial and other vascular cells [20]. It is an extremely potent inhibitor of platelet aggregation and at higher concentrations inhibits primary platelet adhesion [21]. The hypothesis was put forward that PGI_2 secretion by endothelium had a major physiological role in suppressing platelet interaction with the vascular intima [22]. This view, as already indicated, had a big impact on work on the pharmacology of aspirin, leading to the search for a dose of aspirin which would inhibit synthesis of eicosanoids from platelets, while preserving synthesis of PGI_2 by vascular endothelium [8]. Fifteen years of subsequent experience have suggested that the hypothesis is invalid, at least to the extent that complete suppression of PGI_2 synthesis is not sufficient to negate the anti-thrombotic action of high doses of aspirin. PGI_2 also has potent vasodilator activity and it seems likely that this property is of more physiological relevance. Unfortunately the vasodilator action has helped to limit its clinical application because of its tendency, at therapeutically effective doses, to cause profound hypotension [23]. In addition, PGI_2 in solution is unstable, and its plasma half-life is very short. Iloprost is a synthetic prostacyclin which has similar, or greater, potency but is chemically stable in solution at neutral pH. It, also, is a potent inhibitor of platelet aggregation and of primary platelet adhesion *in vitro* [24].

PGI_2 has been shown to preserve platelet function during cardio-pulmonary bypass, and also to limit the fall in platelet number which occurs at the onset of bypass [25]. PGI_2 was also shown to reduce the requirement for heparin during haemodialysis [26]. Iloprost may be particularly useful in limiting platelet interaction with the cardio-pulmonary bypass circuit in patients unsuitable for heparin therapy [27].

Dipyridamole

Dipyridamole is a pyrimido-pyrimidine, a class of compound developed initially as vasodilators. Observation of its apparent platelet inhibitor function was serendipitous. It was applied to a model of platelet micro-aggregate formation in the pial blood vessels of rabbits to prevent vasoconstriction following vascular injury, and found to inhibit platelet microaggregate formation [28]. It was assumed for many years to function as a platelet inhibitor due to its action in inhibiting phosphodiesterase, thereby increasing intra-platelet cyclic AMP levels. More recently, clinical comparisons have cast doubt on whether dipyridamole has any worthwhile anti-thrombotic activity *in vivo* [for example 29] and this has led to a re-evaluation of its activity. At a concentration (200 μM) that inhibits ADP-induced shape-change, dipyridamole did not increase intraplatelet cyclic AMP levels [30]. Other suggestions [31] have been that it stimulates release of PGI_2 by vascular endothelium; inhibits cellular uptake and metabolism of adenosine; and potentiates the action of nitric oxide [32]. Infusion of dipyridamole IV to human volunteers results in a significant increase in plasma concentrations of adenosine [33] which in its turn raises intra-platelet cyclic AMP by stimulating adenylate cyclase. This has been proposed as the explanation for the inhibitory action of dipyridamole on platelets in whole blood, in which red cells can release adenosine, as opposed to the lack of effect in platelet-rich plasma.

The evidence on the action of dipyridamole on primary platelet adhesion is to an extent conflicting. Using blood from volunteers who had taken oral dipyridamole for six days, no effect was shown on platelet deposition to subendothelium in a perfusion device [31]. In contrast, administration of dipyridamole IV to rabbits significantly inhibited platelet deposition on aortas denuded of endothelium by passage of a balloon catheter [34].

Few clinical studies looking at the effect of dipyridamole on platelet interactions with artificial surfaces have been carried out. Dipyridamole was shown to prolong shortened platelet survival in patients with prosthetic heart valves, whereas aspirin was without effect [35]. However, the relevance of shortened platelet survival to vascular injury, platelet deposition and thrombosis is complex and deductions from observations of drug effects on platelet survival to anti-thrombotic activity unreliable. Dipyridamole may have some effect in reducing the thrombo-embolism rate in patients with mechanical prosthetic heart-valves *in situ* who are treated with warfarin [14] though in another study dipyridamole and aspirin in combination did not suppress thromboembolism [36]. Direct comparison of dipyridamole with aspirin in prevention of restenosis following coronary artery bypass grafting has suggested that dipyridamole is without effect in maintenance of graft patency [29] and this study in combination with the lack of other strong evidence of efficacy has lead to a general view that dipyridamole is more-or-less ineffective as a platelet inhibitory agent.

Ticlopidine

The actions of ticlopidine on some aspects of platelet function *in vitro* were first described 17 years ago but its mechanism of action remains unclear. Its main action lies in blocking aggregation in response to ADP [37] and its inhibitory action on other soluble agonists probably relates to its ability to inhibit amplification of platelet activation by released endogenous ADP [38]. In contrast to the effects of aspirin and dipyridamole it markedly prolongs the bleeding time [37]. It does not affect cyclooxygenase, thromboxane synthetase, cAMP phosphodiesterase nor adenylate cyclase. Binding of fibrinogen and von Willebrand factor to glycoprotein IIb/IIIa on the plasma membrane of activated platelets is suppressed in the presence of ticlopidine [39] but this is thought to be the outcome of an action earlier in the process of platelet activation since ticlopidine has not been shown to affect the Gp IIb/IIIa complex directly [39]. Recent studies suggest that ticlopidine inhibits an early step in signal-response coupling following activation of the ADP receptor [40]. Its action is delayed, for reasons which are not understood, the maximum effect taking approximately three days to develop following administration to man.

Evidence of efficacy derived from large-scale clinical trials has been limited, though it has been shown to be at least as effective as aspirin in prevention of cardiovascular events following stroke [41]. It is also effective in prevention of early occlusion of coronary artery bypass grafts [42].

Clinical application in some countries has been limited because it can cause leucopenia.

Inhibitors of thrombin action on platelets

Generation of thrombin is inevitable when blood comes in contact with an artificial surface and thrombin is likely to be a major stimulus to platelet activation in proximity to artificial materials. In whole blood systems it is difficult to disentangle the effects of thrombin inhibitors, what proportion of their action is mediated through an action on platelets and what is dependent on inhibition of thrombin generation.

Heparin

The main action of unfractionated heparin is to bind to antithrombin III and accelerate inhibition of several of the activated coagulation factors, particularly factors IXa, Xa and IIa [43]. Heparin has a complex additional direct effect on platelets, some fractions derived from large molecular forms of heparin causing aggregation of platelets while others are inhibitory [44]. Heparin marginally prolongs the bleeding time when administered to man, [45] though whether by inhibiting thrombin activation of platelets at the wound margin or by some other mechanism is not known.

Heparin has been the essential pharmacological tool which has enabled invasive vascular procedures to be carried out. Renal dialysis and coronary artery bypass surgery require heparinization of the extra-corporeal circuitry to prevent thrombin generation and fibrin formation, and this is dose dependent. The platelet count falls at the onset of cardiopulmonary bypass and to a lesser extent at the onset of dialysis, but as long as coagulation is inhibited platelet activation is not a significant problem. With older dialysers it appeared that adding PGI_2 as an additional antithrombotic measure reduced the requirement for heparin [26] but with later dialysis equipment, suppression of platelet activation with PGI_2 or iloprost had no detectable effect [46]. Heparin bonding to the surface of vascular catheters significantly inhibits deposition of indium-labelled platelets and prevents catheter-tip thrombosis [47] and bonding of heparin to artificial materials reduces platelet deposition [48].

Hirudin

Hirudin is a family of polypeptides found in leeches which have the most powerful anti-thrombin activity so far known. The three main variants which have closely similar activity can now be produced by recombinant technology [49]. Hirudins inhibit thrombin by binding at several recognition sites and blocking the active serine site of the molecule. Because the association rate between hirudin and thrombin is faster than that between thrombin and fibrinogen, hirudin has high potency as an anticoagulant. In addition it inhibits thrombin binding to, and stimulation of, platelets [50].

Though clinical experience with hirudins is limited, experimental systems indicate that they will be at least as effective as heparin in prevention of thrombosis. In an experimental model using a polyethylene arterio-venous shunt, hirudins inhibited formation of platelet-rich thrombi on the artificial surface presumably by limiting thrombin generation and blocking its interaction with platelets [51]. Hirudins have been shown to be more effective than heparin in suppression of clot accretion in rabbits [52].

Synthetic inhibitors of thrombin

Small peptides containing modified forms of the sequence phenylalanine-proline-arginine are effective inhibitors of thrombin, though many of the peptides described are less potent than hirudins. They share with hirudin the ability to inhibit fibrin-bound thrombin, which is inaccessible to antithrombin III and therefore not inhibited by heparins [53]. The efficacy of hirudins and arginine-containing peptides to inhibit platelet-rich thrombus formation has led to a re-appraisal of the role of thrombin in recruiting platelets into forming thrombi and a recognition of its central role [54]. Experimental evidence indicates that a potent peptide Ac-(D)-Phe-Pro-boro Arginine (DuP 714) in addition to its predictable anticoagulant function is a potent inhibitor of platelet-rich thrombus formation in polyvinylchloride arterio-venous shunts in rabbits [55].

Inhibition of adhesin binding

Platelet adhesion to surfaces is dependent on binding of adhesins (adhesive proteins) mainly von Willebrand factor (vWF) and fibronectin, to the surface and to glycoproteins Ib and IIb/IIIa on the membrane of activated platelets. Fibrinogen and thrombospondin are adhesins that bind platelets to each other through Gp IIb/IIIa, which functions as a membrane receptor. Interference with these reactions is a promising route for inhibition of platelet function. Since inhibition of the interaction between fibrinogen and GpIIb/IIIa blocks a final event in platelet aggregation, such inhibitors are likely to prove more effective than agents such as aspirin which block only one pathway of platelet activation.

Peptides containing the arginine-glycine-aspartic acid (RGD) sequence

The adhesive proteins fibrinogen, fibronectin and vWF contain the RGD peptide sequence which is the molecular sub-unit involved in binding to platelet membrane glycoprotein IIb/IIIa. Synthetic RGD-containing peptides inhibit the binding of these proteins in a competitive and reversible manner [56]. In a high shear-rate experimental system, RGD peptides have been shown to inhibit platelet adhesion to subendothelium by 40–70%, depending on the peptide and its concentration [57]. The peptides did not affect platelet adhesion to collagen in a static system [58].

Similar experiments have shown that platelet adhesion to collagen, and subsequent thrombus formation at the surface, is inhibited by the presence of RGD peptides at high shear-rates [58].

The viper venom, echistatin, contains a similar RGD sequence, and has been shown to inhibit platelet aggregation to a range of soluble agonists, as well as inhibit thrombus formation in a model of coronary artery occlusion in dogs [59].

Antibodies to platelet membrane glycoproteins

A complementary approach to competitive blockade of GpIIb/IIIa using RGD peptides has been the use of monoclonal antibodies directed against the membrane glycoprotein which inhibit its function. Various monoclonal antibodies to GpIIb/IIIa have been shown to inhibit binding of adhesive proteins and impair platelet function [60]. Monoclonal antibodies to GPIIb/IIIa impair platelet-surface interaction, probably by interfering with platelet spreading [61]. In experimental systems, monoclonal antibodies to GpIIb/IIIa inhibit thrombosis in extracorporeal arteriovenous shunts in animals [62].

Conclusions

Traditional platelet-inhibitors have proved relatively ineffective in practice, at least partly because of their lack of activity against thrombin-induced platelet activation. The development of agents which specifically inhibit thrombin or block the reaction between adhesive proteins and platelet membrane receptors has emphasised the importance of platelet stimulation by thrombin in thrombogenesis on artificial and damaged vascular surfaces. These newer compounds offer the prospect of more effective inhibition of platelet-mediated thrombosis. However, in clinical practice, platelet interactions with artificial surfaces, including vascular catheters, extracorporeal circuits, cardiac valve prostheses, and synthetic vascular grafts rarely result in significant or clinically relevant problems. Improvements in design, particularly in the reduction of shear stress, have produced devices which, with the use of careful anticoagulation, rarely provoke significant platelet activation. While recent advances in the pharmacology of platelet inhibition have resulted in potent compounds which are highly active in experimental systems, it remains to be determined whether they will yield major gains in clinical practice.

References

1. Portner, P. M., Green, G. F., and Ramasamy, N., 'The blood interface at artificial surfaces within a left ventricular assist system', *Ann. NY Acad. Sci.* 1983, 416: 471–503.
2. Bills, T. K., Smith, J. B., and Silver, M. J., 'Selective release of arachidonic acid from the phospholipids of human platelets in response to thrombin', *J. Clin. Invest.* 1977, 60: 1–8.
3. Gorman, R. R., Bunting. S., and Miller, O. V., 'Modulation of human platelet adenylate cyclase by prostacyclin', *Prostaglandins* 1977, 13: 337–338.
4. Roth, G. J. and Majerus, P. W., 'The mechanism of the effect of aspirin on human platelets. I. Acetylation of a particular fraction protein', *J. Clin. Invest.* 1975, 56: 624–632.
5. Smith, J. G. and Willis, A. L., 'Aspirin selectively inhibits prostaglandin production in human platelets', *Nature (New Biol.)* 1971, 231: 235–237.
6. Weiss, H. J., Tschopp, T. B., and Baumagartner, H. R., 'Impaired interaction (adhesion-aggregation) of platelets with the subendothelium in storage-pool disease and after aspirin ingestion', *N. Engl. J. Med.* 1975, 293: 619–623.
7. Jaffe, E. A. and Weksler, B. B., 'Recovery of endothelial cell prostacyclin production after inhibition by low doses of aspirin', *J. Clin. Invest.* 1979, 63: 532–535.
8. Bochner, F. and Lloyd, J., 'Is there an optimal dose and formulation of aspirin to prevent arterial thrombo-embolism in man?', *Clin. Sci.* 1986, 71: 625–631.
9. Hirsh, H., Salzman, E. W., Harker, L., Fuster, V., Dalen, J. E., Cairns, J. A., and Collins, R., 'Aspirin and other platelet active drugs. Relationship among dose, effectiveness and side effects', *Chest* 1989, 95 (suppl): 12S–18S.
10. Hampton, K. K., Cerletti, C., Loizou, L. A., Bucchi, F., Donati, M. B., Davies, J. A., de Gaetano, G., and Prentice, C. R. M., 'Coagulation, fibrinolytic and platelet function in patients on long-term therapy with aspirin 300 mg or 1,200 mg daily compared with placebo', *Thromb. Haemostas.* 1990, 64: 17–20.
11. Antiplatelet Trialists' Collaboration, 'Secondary prevention of vascular disease by prolonged antiplatelet treatment', *Br. Med. J.* 1988, 296: 320–331.
12. Lam, J. Y. T., Chesebro, J. H., Steele, P. M., Badimon, L., and Fuster, V., 'Is vasospasm related to platelet deposition. Relationship in a porcine preparation of arterial injury *in vivo*', *Circulation* 1987, 75: 243–248.
13. Lindsay, R. M., Ferguson, D., Prentice, C. R. M., Burton, J. A., and McNicol, G. P., 'Reduction of thrombus formation on dialyser membranes by aspirin and RA 233', *Lancet* 1972, 2: 1287–1290.
14. Chesebro, J. H., Fuster, V., McGoon, D. C., *et al.*, 'Trial of combined warfarin plus dipyridamole or aspirin therapy in prosthetic heart valve replacement. Danger of aspirin compared with dipyridamole', *Am. J. Cardiol.* 1983, 51: 1537–1541.
15. Menys, V. C. and Davies J. A., 'Selective inhibition of thromboxane synthetase with dazoxiben – basis of its inhibitor effect on platelet adhesion', *Thromb. Haemostas.* 1983, 49: 96–101.
16. De Clerck, F., Beetens, J., de Chaffoy de Courcelles, D., Freyne, E., and Janssen, P. A., 'R68070: thromboxane A2 synthetase inhibition and thromboxane A2/prostaglandin endoperoxide receptor blockade combined in one molecule – I. Biochemical profile *in vitro*', *Thromb. Haemostas.* 1989, 61: 35–42.
17. De Clerck, F., Beetens, J., Van de Water, A., Vercammen, E., and Janssen, P.A., 'R68070: thromboxane A2 synthetase inhibition and thromboxane A2/prostaglandin endoperoxide

receptor blockade combined in one molecule – II. Pharmacological effects *in vivo* and *ex vivo*', *Thromb. Haemostas.* 1989, 61: 43–49.
18. Fiddler, G. I. and Lumley, P., 'Preliminary clinical studies with thromboxane synthetase inhibitors and thromboxane receptor blockers. A review', *Circulation* 1990, 81 (suppl I): I–69 – I–78.
19. Lane, I. F., Lumley, P., Michael, M. F., Peters, A. M., and McCollum, C. N., 'A specific thromboxane receptor blocking drug, AH23848, reduces platelet deposition on vascular grafts in man', *Thromb. Haemostas.* 1990, 64: 369–373.
20. Moncada, S., Gryglewski, R., Bunting, S., and Vane, J. R., 'An enzyme isolated from arteries transforms prostaglandin endoperoxides to an unstable substance that inhibits platelet aggregation', *Nature* 1976, 263: 663–665.
21. Higgs, E. A., Moncada, S., and Vane, J. R., 'Effect of prostacyclin (PGI_2) on platelet adhesion to rabbit arterial subendothelium', *Prostaglandins* 1978, 16: 17–22.
22. Bunting, S., Moncada, S., and Vane, J. R., 'Prostacyclin-thromboxane A_2 balance', *Br. Med. Bull.* 1983, 39: 271–276.
23. Mitchell, J. R. A., 'Prostacyclin-powerful, yes: but is it useful', *Br. Med. J.* 1983, 287: 1824–1826.
24. Menys, V. C. and Davies, J. A., 'Inhibitory effects of ZK36374, a stable prostacyclin analogue, on adhesion of rabbit platelets to damaged aorta and serotonin release by adherent platelets', *Clin. Sci.* 1983, 65: 149–153.
25. Radegran, K. and Papaconstantinou, C., 'Prostacyclin infusion during cardiopulmonary bypass in man', *Throm. Res.* 1980, 19: 267–270.
26. Weston, M. J., 'Prostacyclin and extracorporeal circulation', *Br. Med. Bull.* 1983, 39: 285–288.
27. Addonizio, V. P., Fisher, C. A., Kappa, J. R., and Ellison, N., 'Prevention of heparin-induced thrombocytopenia during open cardiac surgery with ZK36374 (iloprost)', *Surgery* 1987, 102: 796–807.
28. Emmons, P. R., Harrison, M. J. G., Honour, A. J., and Mitchell, J. R. A., 'Effect of dipyridamole on human platelet behaviour', *Lancet* 1965, 2: 603–606.
29. Brown, B. G., Cukingnan, R. A., De Rouen, T., *et al.*, 'Improved graft patency in patients treated with platelet-inhibiting therapy after coronary bypass surgery', *Circulation* 1985, 72: 138–146.
30. Lam, S. C.-T., Guccione, M. A., Packham, M. A., and Mustard, J. F., 'Effect of cAMP phosphodiesterase inhibitors on ADP-induced shape change, cAMP and nucleoside diphosphokinase activity of rabbit platelets', *Thromb. Haemostas.* 1982, 47: 90–95.
31. Fitzgerald, G. A., 'Dipyridamole', *N. Engl. J. Med.* 1987, 316: 1247–1257.
32. Bult, H., Fret, H. R. L., Jordaens, F. H., and Herman, A. G., 'Dipyridamole potentiates the anti-aggregating and vasodilator activity of nitric oxide', *Eur. J. Pharmacol.* 1991, 199: 1–8.
33. Sollevi, A., Ostergren, J., Fagrell, B., and Hjemdahl, P., 'Theophylline antagonizes cardiovascular responses to dipyridamole in man without affecting increases in plasma adenosine', *Acta Physiol. Scand.* 1984, 121: 165–171.
34. Groves, H. M., Kinlough-Rathbone, R. L., Cazenave, J.-P., Dejana, E., Richardson, M., and Mustard, J. F., 'Effect of dipyridamole and prostacyclin on rabbit platelet adherence *in vitro* and *in vivo*', *J. Lab. Clin. Med.* 1982, 99: 548–558.
35. Harker, L. A. and Slichter, S. J., 'Platelet and fibrinogen consumption in man', *N. Engl. J. Med.* 1972, 287: 999–1005.
36. Brott, W. H., Zajtchuk, R., Bowen, T. E., Davia, J., and Green, D. C., 'Dipyridamole-aspirin as thromboembolic prophylaxis in patients with aortic valve prosthesis: prospective study with the model 2320 Starr-Edwards prosthesis', *J. Thorac. Cardiovasc. Surg.* 1981, 81: 632–635.
37. O'Brien, J. R., Etherington, M.D. and Shuttleworth, R.D., 'Ticlopidine. An antiplatelet drug: effects in human volunteers', *Thromb. Res.* 1978, 13: 245–254.
38. Féliste, R., Delebassée, D., Simon, M. F., Chap, H., Defreyn, G., Vallée, E., Douste-

Blazy, L., and Maffrand, J. P., 'Broad spectrum anti-platelet activity of ticlopidine and PCR 4099 involves the supression of the effects of released ADP', *Thromb. Res.* 1987, 48: 403–415.

39. Di Minno, G., Cerbone, A. M., Mattiolo, P. L., Turco, S., Iovine, C., and Mancini, M., 'Functionally thrombasthenic state in normal platelets following the administration of ticlopidine', *J. Clin. Invest.* 1985, 75: 328–338.
40. Defreyn, G., Gachet, C., Savi, P., Driot, F., Cazenave. J. P., and Maffrand, J. P., 'Ticlopidine and Clopidogrel (SR25990C) selectively neutralise ADP inhibition of PGE_1-activated platelet adenylate cyclase in rats and rabbits', *Thromb. Haemostas.* 1991, 65: 186–190.
41. Hass, W. K., Easton, J. D., Adams, H. P., *et al.*, 'A randomised trial comparing ticlopidine hydrochloride with aspirin for the prevention of stroke in high-risk patients', *N. Engl. J. Med.* 1989, 321: 501–507.
42. Limet, R., David, J. L., Magotteaux, P., *et al.*, 'Prevention of aorto-coronary bypass graft occlusion. Beneficial effect of ticlopidine on early and late patency rates of venous coronary bypass grafts: A double blind study', *J. Thorac. Cardiovasc. Surg.* 1987, 94: 773–783.
43. Hirsh, J., 'Heparin', *N. Engl. J. Med.* 1991, 324: 1565–1574.
44. Salzman, E. W., Rosenberg, R. D., Smith, M. H., Lindon, J. N., and Favreau, L., 'Effect of heparin and heparin fractions on platelet aggregation', *J. Clin. Invest.* 1980, 65: 64–73.
45. Heiden, D., Mielke, C. H., and Rodvien, R., 'Impairment by heparin of primary haemostasis and platelet [14C]5-hydroxytriptamine release', *Br. J. Haematol.* 1977, 36: 427–436.
46. Dibble, J. B., Kalra, P. A., Orchard, M. A., Turney, J. H., and Davies, J. A., 'Prostacyclin and iloprost do not affect action of standard dose heparin on haemostatic function during haemodialysis', *Thromb. Res.* 1988, 49: 385–392.
47. Hoar, P. F., Wilson, R. M., Mangano, D. T., Avery, G. J., Szarnicki, R. J. and Hill, J. D., 'Heparin bonding reduces thrombogenicity of pulmonary-artery catheters', *N. Engl. J. Med.* 1981, 305: 993–995.
48. Ito, Y., Iguchi, Y., and Imanishi, Y., 'Synthesis and non-thrombogenicity of heparinoid polyurethaneureas', *Biomaterials* 1992, 13: 131–135.
49. Märki, W. E. and Wallis, R. B., 'The anticoagulant and antithrombotic properties of hirudins', *Thromb. Haemostas.* 1990, 64: 344–348.
50. Markwardt, F., 'Development of hirudin as an antithrombotic agent', *Sem. Thromb. Haemostas.* 1989, 15: 269–282.
51. Markwardt, F., Kaiser, B., and Novac, G., 'Studies on antithrombotic effects of recombinant hirudin', *Thromb. Res.* 1989, 54: 377–388.
52. Agnelli, G., Pascucci, C., Cosmi, B., and Nenci, G. G., 'The comparative effects of recombinant hirudin (CGP39393) and standard heparin on thrombus growth in rabbits', *Thromb. Haemostas.* 1990, 63: 204–207.
53. Weitz, J. I., Hudoba, M., Massel, D., Maraganore, J., and Hirsh, J., 'Clot-bound thrombin is protected from inhibition by heparin-antithrombin III but is susceptible to inactivation by antithrombin III-independent inhibitors', *J. Clin. Invest.* 1990, 86: 385–391.
54. Hanson, S. R. and Harker, L. A., 'Interruption of acute platelet-dependent thrombosis by the synthetic antithrombin D-phenylalanyl-L-prolyl-L-arginyl chloromethyl ketone', *Proc. Natl. Acad. Sci. USA* 1988, 85: 3184–3188.
55. Knabb, R. M., Kettner, C. A., Timmermans, P. B. M. W. M., and Reilly, T. M., '*In vivo* characterization of a new synthetic thrombin inhibitor', *Thromb. Haemostas.* 1992, 67: 56–59.
56. Plow, E. F., Pierschbacher, M. D., Ruoslahti, E., Marguerie, G. A., and Ginsberg, M. H., 'The effect of Arg-Gly-Asp-containing peptides on fibrinogen and von Willebrand factor binding to platelets', *Proc. Natl. Acad. Sci. USA* 1985, 82: 8057–8061.
57. Lawrence, J. B., Kramer, W. S., McKeown, L. P., Williams, S. B., and Gralnick, H. R., 'Arginine-glycine-aspartic acid- and fibrinogen chain carboxyterminal peptides inhibit

platelet adherence to arterial subendothelium at high wall shear rates', *J. Clin. Invest.* 1990, 86: 1715–1722.

58. Fressinaud, E., Girma, J. P., Sadler, J. E., Baumgartner, H. R., and Meyer, D., 'Synthetic RGDS-containing peptides of von Willebrand factor inhibit platelet adhesion to collagen', *Thromb. Haemostas.* 1990, 64: 589–593.
59. Shebuski, R. J., Ramjit, D. R., Sitko, G. R., Lumma, P. K., and Garsky, V.M., 'Prevention of canine coronary artery thrombosis with echistatin, a potent inhibitor of platelet aggregation from the venom of the viper, echis carinatus', *Thromb. Haemostas.* 1990, 64: 576–581.
60. Coller, B. S., Peerschke, E. I., Scudder, L. E., and Sullivan, C. A., 'A murine monoclonal antibody that completely blocks the binding of fibrinogen to platelets produces a thrombasthenic-like state in normal platelet and binds to glycoprotein IIb and/or IIIa', *J. Clin. Invest.* 1983, 72: 325–328.
61. Lawrence, J. B. and Gralnick, H. R., 'Monoclonal antibodies to the glycoprotein IIb-IIIa epitopes involved in adhesive protein binding: effects on platelet spreading and ultrastructure on human arterial subendothelium', *J. Lab. Clin. Med.* 1987, 109: 495–503.
62. Hanson, S. R., Pareti, F. I., Ruggeri, Z. M., Marzec, U. M., Kunicki, T. J., Montgomery, R. R., Zimmerman, T. S., and Harker, L. A., 'Effects of monoclonal antibodies against the platelet glycoprotein IIb/IIIa complex on thrombosis and hemostasis in the baboon', *J. Clin. Invest.* 1988, 81: 149–158.

PART TWO

Platelet surface interactions: cellular and rheological aspects

5. The role of hemodynamics on the cellular responses

Y.F. MISSIRLIS
Biomedical Engineering Laboratory, University of Patras, Patras, Greece

Introduction

Blood and its elements experience during their life-time in the circulation a great variety of rheological conditions depending on their spatio-temporal coordinates during each cardiac cycle.

Every blood cell (erythrocyte, leucocyte, platelet) will be displaced with varying velocity and acceleration, during each infinitesimal time period, dt, and may move along a streamline usually interacting with other cells, proteins, or the wall surface.

Each cell during this time, dt, may be deformed, according to its intrinsic mechanical properties; such deformation may be associated with important changes in the functional dynamics of the cells, both internal and external, such as:

- Membrane pore openings with increased permeability of small ions
- Conformational changes with exposure of previously unexposed functional groups of membrane glycoproteins
- Release (or uptake) of a multitude of substances from the cytoplasm (free or within organells)
- Metabolic alterations, *et al.*

Under normal, healthy circulatory conditions such events as described previously may be within the reversible limits set by the homeostatic processes. However, when trauma, disease or other abnormality is encountered these events may become very energetic leading to transient or permanent changes involving a multitude of interactions and consequences, such as thrombus formation, embolization, atherosclerosis *et al.*

When in addition an artificial surface comes into contact with the flowing blood, either temporarily or permanently, more events, stemming from the artificial surface interference, interplay with those already mentioned resulting usually in dramatic consequences.

In this paper an overview of the various techniques which have been utilized in order to assess the behaviour of blood cells and in particular of platelets in contact with surfaces under flow conditions will be attempted.

Y. F. Missirlis and J.-L. Wautier (eds.), The Role of Platelets in Blood-Biomaterial Interactions, 61–67.

Fluid dynamic considerations of blood

Blood flows within the cardiovascular system (or in extracorporeal circuits) due to pressure differences and boundary wall movements which are generated in the cardiovascular system, or by artificial assist pumps.

The actual pressure-velocity relationships vary tremendously from the ventricles to capillaries and the relative importance of the intrinsic properties of the flowing cells is different in the large vessels from that in the microcirculation.

However a few approximations, which follow, will provide us with some indicative numbers relating to the forces that the cells experience.

a) For steady flow of a Newtonian fluid (i.e. plasma) through a long cylindrical tube of constant cross-sectional area and rigid walls the relationship between the velocity profile in the fully developed flow and the driving pressure is:

$$V_z = \frac{\Delta P}{L}\frac{R^2}{4n}\left[1 - (\frac{r}{R})^2\right] = 2V_0\left[1 - (\frac{r}{R})^2\right]$$

where V_z is the axial velocity, V_0 the mean velocity, R the vessel radius, ΔP the pressure drop, L the length of the vessel, n the viscosity of the fluid.

This parabolic velocity profile is valid for relatively low flow rates (Re $<$ 2100) which is the case in almost all healthy human blood vessels[1].

For the Newtonian fluids in laminar (low flow rate) flow each fluid layer is sliding past each other thus generating a *shear stress* (loss of energy), τ, which is

$$\tau = n\frac{dV_z}{dr} = n\dot{\gamma}$$

where $\dot{\gamma}$ is the *shear rate* (which measures how rapidly the fluid layers are sliding past each other).

At the vessel centerline the shear rate is zero (therefore the shear stress is also zero). The maximum value of shear is exhibited at the wall ($r = R$) and it is

$$\dot{\gamma}_w = \frac{4V_0}{R}$$

and

$$\tau_w = \frac{4nV_0}{R}.$$

[1] More complex relations are found in classical text books [1, 2] for pulsatile flow in cylindrical distensible vessels.

With plasma viscosity of 1.2 centipoise = 1.2 mPa.s = $1.2.10^{-2}$ dyn/cm^2.s the wall shear rates (time average values, because of pulsatility) in the blood vessels vary from zero in regions of stasis to 10^5 s^{-1} in high flow arterioles and in some prosthetic heart valves [3]. The corresponding wall shear stress, therefore, would be from zero to 1.2 mPa.s $\times$ 10^5 s^{-1} = 1.2×10^2 Pa = 1.2×10^3 dyn/cm^2.

Whole blood does not have a constant viscosity (rather called *apparent viscosity* because of its dispersive character). In situations of stasis the *relative viscosity* (compared to that of plasma) can reach the value of 100, whereas for shear rates greater than about 500 s^{-1} the viscosity is approximately constant to values of about 3–4. Under such conditions the blood viscosity is dependent on the hematocrit. Therefore in order to calculate the shear stress from the shear rate, or *vice versa*, especially at very low flow rates, one needs know the apparent viscosity of the blood for the particular situation.

Arteries respond to changing flow regimes by remodeling the diameter to keep the wall shear stress around 15 dyn/cm^2 [4]. Other estimates give values from 25–110 dyn/cm^2, the larger values for the small arterioles [5].

Mass transport

The flowing plasma proteins and blood cells move axially and radially in a complex manner depending on the local shear rate which may change due to pulsatility, geometrical changes and associated secondary flows. The access of these elements (proteins, cells) to the wall or to a blood contacting biomaterial surface in general occurs by molecular diffusion or by fluid convection.

The mass transport will be mainly due to convection as the diffusion in liquids is too slow (diffusivity coefficients 10^{-5} to 10^{-8} cm^2/s). If there was only fully developed laminar steady flow the access to the wall would be very slow (by diffusion) as the fluid velocity is only axial. Any disturbance (curvature, wall abnormalities, expansions or contractions of the cross-sectional areas, and of course pulsatility) would generate radial velocities and thus would greatly increase the mass transport to the wall.

Cell behaviour in shear flow

Cells that find themselves in a shear field will be deformed, their membrane being stretched or compressed or bended or twisted, they will rotate (in red blood cells their membrane rotates, "tank treads" around the cytoplasm), and they may collide with other cells or particles, the rate of collision depending on the concentration, particle volume and relative speeds.

All these events can take place separately or alltogether. Colliding cells may form aggregates. Aggregate formation depends on the frequency of collision (which depends linearly on the local shear rate) and the effectiveness of the collision (how well the colliding cells stick together) [6]. Apparently disaggregating forces also increase as the shear rate increases.

The degree of distortion of a cell in a shear field depends both on the stress level and the time of exposure to the particular stress. The cells can tolerate extremely high shear stress if exposure time is short enough. Platelets, leucocytes and erythrocytes have quite different thresholds of combinations of stress level-exposure times [7]. For example, for exposure times of tens of seconds (0–100 s) erythrocytes can tolerate shear stresses of up to 2000 dyn/cm^2 without lysis, while leucocytes can withstand only 200 dyn/cm^2 and platelets from 200–300 dyn/cm^2. On the contrary for exposure times of 0.1 to 1 ms, erythrocytes will remain unhemolysed for shear stresses up to 5000 dyn/cm^2 while platelets are sturdier being lysed at stresses 20–30.000 dyn/cm^2 [7].

Lysis of erythrocytes releases ADP which is a potent factor or triggering platelet aggregation. However of particular importance may be the cellular changes, such as release reactions, conformational changes, mechanical alterations, which occur under sublytic stress exposure and may have direct influence on the activation and aggregation of platelets and leucocytes.

One other characteristic of the effect of shear on cellular activities is a synergistic effect produced by erythrocytes on platelets. In flow, the rotation of individual erythrocytes generates local fluid motion enabling the platelets which are found in the neighborhood to "diffuse" to a greater extent, augmenting their rate of arrival at the wall for example [8]. Such an augmentation is very important at high shear rates, and up to a hematocrit of about 40%, but negligible at low shear rates.

The question remains, especially in designing artificial organs, what is the optimum shear rate that would maintain sufficient blood flow, would not destroy or activate cells, would disaggregate formed aggregates and detach weakly adherent cells from the wall.

Except blood cells the endothelium is also affected by the shear field (as well as the endothelium-cell attachments). The morphology of the endothelial cells, the expression of certain factors on their surface and even their integrity may be compromised in regions of high flow [9, 10].

Selected examples

Wurzinger and Schmid-Schönbein [11] used a Couette viscometer (gap between two cylinders) to generate shear rates up to 214.000 s^{-1} with cell exposure time from 7 to 700 ms. They found a linear increase in the amount of β-TG released with time at various stress levels, the same for lactic dehydrogenase but could not find a decisive clue of the shear forces on the biological effects on platelets.

McIntire *et al.* [12] used two different apparatuses to subject cells to shear stress. A cone and plate Ferranti-Shirley viscometer, where the whole sample experienced the same constant stress of 150 dyn/cm^2 for 1 min (either platelet rich plasma or leucocyte suspension). Also a parallel plate flow apparatus, the one plate being a glass slide with human umbilical vein endothelial cells culture-seeded on it, was used where steady flows from 0 to 24 dyn/cm^2 (at the wall) or pulsatile flows 8–12 dyn/cm^2 at 1H_z could be produced. Their results showed that platelets, leucocytes and endothelial cells all appear to be sensitive to stress-induced activation of arachidonic acid metabolism. Platelets increased synthesis of the 12-hydroperoxy-eicosatetraenoic acid (12-HPETE) but very little thromboxane B_2.

Production of 12-HPETE under stress induced production of leukotriene B_4 (LTB_4) which induces PMN leucocyte aggregation and degranulation. Production of PGI_2 increased linearly over the applied shear stress and the physiologically pulsatile flow increased the production 2.4 times for the same mean stress. The implications that mechanical stresses may be important on intracellular protein synthesis and cell growth are obvious.

In a Couette rotational viscometer [13] at shear stresses of 150 and 300 dyn/cm^2, sheared for 5 min erythrocytes liberated ADP (without lysis, of course, at this low stress) and furthermore it was found that in citrated platelet rich plasma sheared at 50 dyn/cm^2 for 5 min into which washed erythrocytes were added increased the aggregation of platelets.

In an annular flow system, one cylindrical surface being the subendothelium of a rabbit aorta, citrated blood recirculated permitting platelets to interact with the wall at shear rates of 800 s^{-1} and 2600 s^{-1} [14] for 5 min. The purpose was to examine the role of the platelet membrane receptor GPIIb-IIIa and the adhesive proteins known to bind to it in mediating the interaction of platelets with the subendothelium. At the high shear rate (2600 s^{-1}) it was concluded that fibrinogen is not involved in either GPIIb-IIIa mediated platelet adhesion or thrombus formation. The data were inconclusive regarding the role of fibronectin. GPIIb-IIIa is an important receptor for adhesion under static conditions but may be less important under flow conditions, under which when the other platelet receptor for fibronectin, GPIb is suggested to be involved [15]. The von Willebrand factor (vWF) appeared to be the most likely adhesive protein involved in GPIIb-IIIa mediated platelet adhesion and thrombus formation. The limited data for the shear rate of 800 s^{-1} suggested that the role of the receptor GPIIb-IIIa and the adhesive ligands may be different at this shear rate.

Discussion

This short overview underlines the complexity of events that take place in the interaction of blood and its components with surfaces, the importance of flow considerations and the need to design experiments which incorporate the useful pieces of information derived from very interesting research experiments till now.

It is interesting to note the multiplicity of reports where various flow systems have been used, different shear rates and times of exposure, different species, anticoagulants, measured variables [16], antibodies to specific receptors etc.

Is there a useful picture emerging by putting all this information from *in vitro* experiments together? Are the most relevant parameters taken into account in carrying out experiments? Are the coupling effects considered and have methodologies been proposed to evaluate, for each of the various situations that the blood elements find themselves, the pertinent parameters?

In trying to answer these and similar questions one should consider how to come up with standardization concepts which would not inhibit the innovative approach or "blacklist" different methodologies but on the other hand should make comparisons, evaluations and reaffirmations in different laboratories less cumbersome.

One should bear in mind that it is impossible to take all important factors into account (someone will always be missing) and also that even the best thought and executed experiment would give an approximate picture of the real events.

As was said before, for example many experiments are done at well controlled shear rates of 5, 30, 150, 800, 2000 s^{-1}, which are estimated to be physiological. However peak wall shear rates in pulsatile large arteries, or in prosthetic heart valves, or in stenotic arteries may reach several thousands to hundreds of thousands s^{-1} [3, 14].

A simple perfusion system where blood (or other fluid) flow controlled by a syringe pump through one or more capillaries or small diameter tubes with a steady laminar flow generating wall shear rates of 0 to 4000 s^{-1} has been used to evaluate many parameters in protein adsorption, platelet adhesion/activation, coagulation and complement systems [17–19].

Recently we developed a software program to control the syringe pump in this system in order to generate unsteady flows (pulsatile and other flow patterns). It is hoped that such simple but well controlled experiments will minimize the ambiguities of the investigations of blood-material interactions.

References

1. Fung, Y.C., *Biodynamics: Circulation.* Springer-Verlag, New York, 1984.
2. Lightfoot, E. N., *Transport Phenomena and Living Systems.* John Wiley, New York, 1974.
3. *Guidelines for Blood-Material Interactions.* Report of the N.H.L.B.I. Working Group. NIH Publication No 85–2185, 1985.
4. Giddens, D. P., Zarins, C. K., and Glagov, S., 'Response of arteries to near-wall fluid dynamic behavior', *Appl. Mech. Rev.* 1990, 43: S98–S102.
5. Schmid-Schönbein, H., Fischer, T., Driessen, G., and Rieger, H., 'Microcirculation', in: *Quantitative Cardiovascular Studies*, Hwang, N. H. C., Gross, D. R., and Patel, D. J. (Eds.), University Park Press, Battimore, 1979.
6. Jen, C. I. and McIntire, L. V., 'Characteristics of shear-inducted aggregation in whole blood', *J. Lab. Clin. Med.* 1984, 103: 115.

7. Hellums, J. D. and Hardwick, P. A., 'Response of platelets to shear stress-a review', in: *The Rheology of Blood, Blood Vessels and Associated Tissue*, Gross, D.R. and Hwang, N.H.C. (Eds.), Sijthoff and Noordhoff, Rockville, 1981.
8. Keller, K. H., 'Effect of fluid shear on mass transport in flowing blood', *Feder. Proc.* 1971, 30: 1591.
9. Fry, D. L., 'Acute vascular endothelial changes associated with increased blood velocity gradients', *Circ. Res.* 1968, 22: 165.
10. Dewey, C. F., Bussolari, S. R., Gimbrone, M. A., and Davies, P. F., 'The dynamic response of vascular endothelial cells to fluid shear stress', *J. Biomech. Eng.* 1981, 103: 177.
11. Wurzinger, L. J. and Schmid-Schönbein, H., 'Surface abnormalities and conduit characteristics as a cause of blood trauma in artificial internal organs', in: *Blood in Contact with Natural and Artificial Surfaces*, Leonard, E.F., Turrito, V.I. and Vroman, L., *Annals N.Y.A.S.* 1987, 516: 316.
12. McIntire, L. V. *et al.*, 'The effect of fluid mechanical stress on cellular arachidonic acid metabolism', in: *Blood in Contact with Natural and Artificial Surfaces*, Leonard, E. F., Turrito, V. T., and Vroman, L., *Annals N.Y.A.S.* 1987, 516: 513.
13. Reimers, R. C., Sutera, S. P., and Loist, J. H., 'Potentiation by red blood cells of shear-induced platelet aggregation', *Blood* 1984, 64: 1200–1206.
14. Weiss, H. J. *et al.*, 'Fibrinogen-independent platelet adhesion and thrombus formation on subendothelium mediated by GPIIb-IIIa complex at high shear rate', *J. Clin. Invest.* 1989, 83: 288–297.
15. Sixma, J. J. *et al.*, 'Vessel wall proteins adhesive for platelets', *J. Biomater. Sci. Polymer Edn.* 1991, 3: 17–26.
16. Olijslager, J., *The development of test devices for the study of blood material interactions.* Ph.D. Thesis, Delft University Press, 1982.
17. Mulvihill, J. N. *et al.*, 'The use of monoclonal antibodies of human platelet membrane GPIIb-IIIa to quantitate platelet deposition on artificial surfaces', *Thromb. Haemostas.* 1987, 58: 724–731.
18. Poot, A. *et al.*, 'Platelet deposition in a capillary perfusion model', *Biomaterials* 1988, 9: 126–132.
19. Missirlis, Y. F. and Michanetzis, G., 'Measurement of platelet adhesion, released β-TG and generated FP-A using whole anticoagulated blood at flow conditions', submitted, 1992.

6. Platelet adhesion to surfaces

J. N. MULVIHILL and J.-P. CAZENAVE
INSERM U.311, Biologie et Pharmacologie des Interactions du Sang avec les Vaisseaux et les Biomatériaux, Centre Régional de Transfusion Sanguine, Strasbourg, France

Adhesion of blood platelets to an injured vessel wall is the first and crucial step in the haemostatic process. Platelet adhesion is also the first step in the development of pathological thrombi when subendothelial structures are exposed to the circulation following endothelial damage and detachment or rupture of an atherosclerotic plaque [1] and the interaction of platelets with disrupted atherosclerotic lesions is the most frequent cause of thrombotic occlusion of coronary and cerebral arteries. Thrombosis of vascular implants and extracorporeal circulatory systems is likewise triggered by platelet adhesion to artificial surfaces in contact with flowing blood [2].

The sequence of events leading to formation of a haemostatic plug or platelet-fibrin thrombus may be depicted as follows [3, 4]. Firstly, a zone of vascular injury or protein coated artificial surface is recognized by platelets which contact and adhere, becoming activated and changing shape from smooth discs to spiny spheres. Secondly, platelet activation is accompanied by secretion of their granule contents, release of adhesive membrane receptors. This leads to platelet spreading on the surface and interplatelet bridging, with formation of surface bound aggregates. Thirdly, thrombin generation causes further platelet activation and transformation of fibrinogen into polymeric fibrin, thus enmeshing the platelets in a secondary haemostatic plug or platelet-fibrin thrombus more resistant to the shear stress of blood flow.

Haemodynamic factors

Blood flow rate is one of the major factors determining platelet adhesion. The annular perfusion chamber of Baumgartner and Haudenschildt [5] first made it possible to study *in vitro* the adhesion of platelets from flowing blood onto the subendothelium of blood vessels, while later development of a flat perfusion chamber [6] and of capillary perfusion systems [7, 8] allowed this type of experiment to be extended to artificial surfaces coated with purified proteins or cultured vessel wall cells. In general, adhesion increases with wall shear rate. This phenomenon arises from the inhomogeneous distribution of cells in flowing blood, the larger red cells being concentrated in the centre of the stream and the smaller platelets forced aside towards the vessel walls [9]. Local concentrations of platelets are thus higher in the vicinity of the wall

Y. F. Missirlis and J.-L. Wautier (eds.), The Role of Platelets in Blood-Biomaterial Interactions, 69–80.

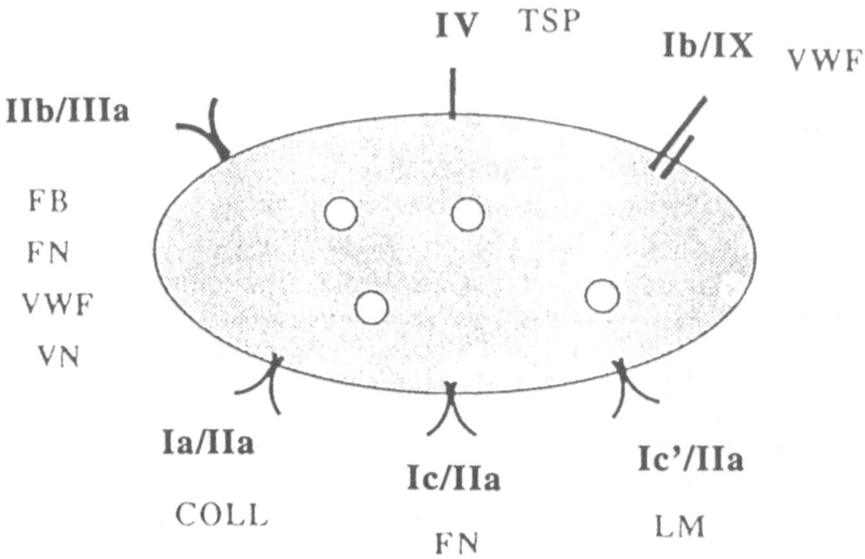

Figure 1. Adhesive proteins and platelet membrane receptors involved in platelet interactions with subendothelium and blood contacting artificial surfaces. FB: fibrinogen, FN: fibronectin, VWF: von Willebrand factor, VN: vitronectin, COLL: collagen, TSP: thrombospondin, LM: laminin.

and this effect is enhanced with increasing shear force. Red cell concentration and rotational motion also influence lateral platelet transport, increased lateral diffusion being observed under conditions of higher haematocrit or greater red cell size and rigidity [10].

Adhesive interactions of platelets with surfaces

On contact with the wall of a natural or artificial vessel, adhesive interactions of platelets are governed by physical factors such as the shear forces and by the presence of adhesive molecules on the exposed subendothelial matrix or protein coated artificial surface. Platelets possess membrane receptors for adhesive proteins present in plasma and/or subendothelium (Table 1, Figure 1). Since the affinity of platelets for an adhesive protein must be sufficiently high to withstand detachment by shear forces, at different flow rates different proteins play a predominant role in platelet adhesion, spreading and formation of surface bound aggregates.

TABLE 1
Adhesive proteins and platelet membrane receptors involved in platelet interactions with subendothelium and blood contacting artificial surfaces

Platelet Membrane Receptors	Adhesive Proteins	Localization
GP Ia-IIa	Collagen	Subendothelium
GP Ib-IX	vWF, fibronectin	Plasma, platelet α-granules, subendothelium
GP Ic-IIa	Fibronectin	Plasma, platelet α-granules, subendothelium
GP Ic′-IIa, 67 kDa receptor	Laminin	Subendothelium
GP IIb-IIIa	Fibrinogen	Plasma, platelet α-granules, artificial surfaces
	vWF, fibronectin	Plasma, platelet α-granules, subendothelium
	Vitronectin	Plasma, artificial surfaces
GP IV	Thrombospondin	Platelet α-granules

Von Willebrand factor

At wall shear rates above 500 s^{-1}, von Willebrand Factor (vWF) is essential for normal platelet adhesion to subendothelium [11]. This multimeric glycoprotein (240,000 Da subunits), synthesized in endothelial cells and megakaryocytes, is present in platelet α-granules and plasma as multimers ranging in size from 1 to 12 million Da and in the subendothelial extracellular matrix [12–14]. The primary receptor for vWF on platelets is the membrane glycoprotein (GP) complex GP Ib-IX. Three distinct polypeptide chains (GP Ibα, GP Ibβ and GP IX) are involved in this receptor system, the vWF binding site being localized on a 45,000 Da fragment of GP Ibα [15]. On vWF, the domain which interacts with GP Ib consists of two sequences of 15 amino acids on either side of a 180 amino acid loop closed by a disulphide bond [16].

GP Ib-IX is already expressed on the plasma membrane of non activated platelets. Its adhesive interaction with vWF is however observed only when vWF is bound to a surface, treated with neuraminidase or in the presence of botrocetin or ristocetin. Although the nature of the change in vWF under these conditions is as yet unknown, the additional requirement for minimal shear forces ($> 650\ s^{-1}$) has led to the hypothesis of shear induced conformational changes in GP Ib and/or vWF which could trigger a specific interaction between these two molecules [17]. The important functional role of this receptor-ligand interaction in the arterial circulation is widely documented. Congenital abnormalities of GP Ib (Bernard-Soulier syndrome) or vWF (von Willebrand disease) are responsible for severe bleeding disorders [18, 19], while defective GP Ib binding to vWF in the presence of anti-GP Ib or anti-vWF antibodies results in markedly reduced platelet adhesion [20, 21]. vWF also binds to activated platelets via the fibrinogen receptor GP IIb-IIIa. This secondary interaction of GP IIb-IIIa with adhesive proteins present on the vessel wall or secreted from platelet α-granules, in particular fibrinogen, vWF and fibronectin, is necessary for platelet spreading [22] and the stabilization of surface bound aggregates.

Fibronectin

Fibronectin is a dimeric or multimeric protein (220,000 Da subunits) present in plasma, platelet α-granules and the subendothelial extracellular matrix. At low shear rates ($< 500\ s^{-1}$), where the interaction of platelet GP Ib with vWF is of lesser importance, fibronectin plays a primary role in platelet adhesion to subendothelium [11]. Platelets possess a specific receptor for fibronectin, the integrin complex GP Ic-IIa. In a static system, this receptor has been shown to mediate adhesion of non activated platelets to surface bound fibronectin [23], but under flow conditions GP Ic-IIa does not appear to be involved in adhesion and GP Ib has been proposed as the principal receptor for platelet adhesion to fibronectin under flow [11]. In common with other adhesive proteins, fibronectin also recognizes the GP IIb-IIIa complex expressed on activated platelets [24]. Once contact activation has occurred, fibronectin will therefore contribute together with vWF and fibrinogen to platelet surface spreading and interplatelet bridging mediated by GP IIb-IIIa. A further contribution to these stabilizing interactions may be afforded by vitronectin. This adhesive protein, present in plasma and associated with platelets, recognizes the activation dependent GP IIb-IIIa complex and in view of its high affinity for glass could play a role in platelet adhesion to artificial surfaces [25].

Collagen

Fibrillar collagen is a major and highly thrombogenic component of vascular subendothelium. Platelet adhesion to subendothelial collagen, mainly types I and III, is particularly important under low or moderate shear forces where vWF interactions are no longer predominant and leads to rapid platelet activation, secretion and surface phase aggregation [1]. Initial attachment of non activated platelets to collagen fibres is Mg^{2+} dependent and occurs via the membrane integrin receptor GP Ia-IIa [26]. Platelets deficient in this receptor show impaired adhesion not only to collagen but also to subendothelium and fail to respond to collagen induced aggregation [27, 28]. Recent studies have demonstrated that the binding site for GP Ia-IIa is located within the $\alpha 1$(I)–CB3 fragment of the collagen molecule and concerns a four amino acid sequence asp-gly-glu-ala (DGEA), whereas further reactions giving rise to platelet activation and aggregation appear to depend on a distinct collagen determinant separate from the GP Ia-IIa recognition site [29, 30]. Hence the proposition of a two-step, two-site model of platelet interaction with fibrillar collagen. The initial direct adhesion of platelets to collagen fibres by high affinity binding of GP Ia-IIa to the DGEA sequence would bring into close proximity a second membrane receptor of lower affinity and it is the binding of this second receptor to an adjacent collagen determinant, possibly through multiple linked interactions, which would lead to activation, secretion and subsequent aggregation of platelets. This hypothesis does not exclude indirect adhesive reactions via intermediary bridging molecules. Proteins such as vWF and fibronectin, which bind to both collagen and one or more platelet surface receptors, may be expected to contribute to early adhesive interactions [31] and in particular once activation has occurred to further spreading and anchoring of platelet thrombi on the collagen fibres.

Laminin

Laminin is a basement membrane glycoprotein (~ 780,000 Da) known to promote cell attachment and migration. Under static conditions, adhesion of platelets to laminin occurs without their activation [32] and is mediated by the integrin receptor GP Ic′-IIa [33]. In a flow system, subendothelial laminin appears to play a significant role in platelet adhesion at relatively low wall shear rates (800 s^{-1}), the interaction in this case being dependent on a 67,000 Da cell surface receptor and on the laminin A chain sequence ile-lys-val-ala-val [34].

Microfibrils

Microfibrils associated with subendothelial elastin and basement membrane constitute yet another potentially thrombogenic component of the vessel wall. In the presence of plasma vWF, platelets adhere to microfibrils through binding of vWF to its membrane receptor GP Ib and to a 97,000 Da protein of the microfibrillar structure, activation then being triggered by a second microfibrillar site which has been characterized to date as a 120,000 Da glycoprotein similar to thrombospondin [35]. However, the relative importance of vWF mediated platelet interactions with microfibrils in platelet adhesion to the vascular subendothelium *in vivo* remains to be established.

Fibrinogen and fibrin

Fibrinogen is an essential requirement for platelet aggregation induced by agonists such as ADP or thrombin, where its interaction with the membrane receptor GP IIb-IIIa expressed on activated platelets allows the formation of interplatelet bridges [4]. The major role of fibrinogen in platelet adhesion at sites of vessel injury is thus in the secondary development of surface bound aggregates. A significant contribution from direct adhesion of platelets to fibrinogen coated surfaces may nevertheless be expected in the case of vascular implants, since foreign materials in contact with flowing blood commonly exhibit preferential adsorption of fibrinogen relative to other plasma proteins and adsorbed fibrinogen enhances platelet adhesion to the majority of these surfaces [36–39]. Direct interaction of platelets with fibrin will likewise be important in the growth of platelet-fibrin thrombi.

A major constituent of plasma and platelet α-granules, the fibrinogen molecule (340,000 Da) is composed of three pairs of non identical polypeptide chains (Aα, Bβ and γ) linked by a series of disulphide bonds [40]. One platelet receptor recognition domain is situated on the carboxy-terminal segment of the γ chain within residues 400 to 411. The α chain bears two further recognition sites (residues 95 to 98 and 572 to 575), both of which contain the sequence arg-gly-asp (RGD) common to a wide range of adhesive proteins including vWF, fibronectin and vitronectin [41]. Ligand specificity is thought to be conserved by the unique γ chain domain. Optimal binding of platelets in aggregation and other adhesive reactions is obtained in combination with the two α chain domains, one fibrinogen molecule bridging two platelets being under these conditions trivalent with respect to each platelet.

The platelet receptor for fibrinogen, an activation dependent complex formed from two membrane glycoproteins GP IIb and GP IIIa, belongs to the integrin family of cell adhesion molecules [42]. Integrins are heterodimeric non covalent complexes of a common β chain and a variable α chain. In the presence of physiological calcium concentrations, the two transmembrane glycoproteins GP IIb and GP IIIa are assembled in 1:1 stoichiometry into the heterodimer GP IIb-IIIa. This complex is the most abundant surface receptor on platelets with about 50,000 copies per cell on the non activated plasma membrane and a pool of similar order in internal membrane systems which is expressed when activation is accompanied by secretion [43]. Binding of fibrinogen to GP IIb-IIIa is specific, Ca^{2+} dependent and fulfils 1:1 stoichiometry [44]. At a molecular level, the dodecapeptide of the fibrinogen γ chain (γ 400–411) appears to interact specifically with GP IIbα, while GP IIIa contains a 63 amino acid sequence with strong affinity for RGD peptides such as those of the fibrinogen α chain [43]. Congenital deficiency of GP IIb-IIIa leads to a bleeding disorder known as Glanzmann's thrombasthenia. Platelets from these patients do not bind fibrinogen [45], nor do they respond to ADP or thrombin induced aggregation or in clot retraction tests [46]. GP IIb-IIIa is further involved in binding of vWF, fibronectin and vitronectin to thrombin stimulated platelets [47–49]. Monoclonal antibodies against the GP IIb-IIIa complex [44] interfere with platelet spreading and thrombus formation *ex vivo* and inhibit platelet dependent occlusion of coronary arteries in dogs and Dacron vascular grafts in baboons [50, 51]. Similar results have been reported using synthetic peptide analogues of the fibrinogen γ chain recognition domain [52] and RGD peptides [53], while an antibody to the γ chain sequence (γ 385–411) was effective in blocking platelet interaction with fibrinogen adsorbed to an artificial polymer surface [54]. Current work in this field is aimed at the development of new antithrombotic agents directed against the binding site on platelet GP IIb-IIIa for fibrinogen, vWF and other adhesive proteins.

Exposition of the functional membrane receptor GP IIb-IIIa requires platelet activation. This transformation from a non binding to a binding mode probably involves conformational modifications and/or partial cleavage of GP IIb, GP IIIa or neighbouring membrane components, which would enable access of bulky adhesive macromolecules to the receptor site [4]. Platelet activation also induces cis-translocation and clustering of GP IIb-IIIa complexes [55]. In perfusion studies of platelet interaction with fibrin and fibrinogen coated glass, adhesion was found to be mediated by GP IIb-IIIa and in the case of the fibrinogen surface to involve an activation linked conformational change of the glycoprotein complex [56]. Densities of adherent platelets were higher on fibrin than on fibrinogen coatings. However, there appeared to be a lesser tendency to platelet activation and aggregation on the fibrin surface, a point which could be relevant to the role of platelet adhesion to fibrin in thrombus and haemostatic plug formation.

Thrombospondin

Thrombospondin is a high molecular weight protein (420,000 Da) secreted from the α-granules of activated platelets [57]. Following its release, thrombospondin binds to the platelet membrane via the glycoprotein receptor GP IV and may further interact with other adhesive proteins present at the surface of platelets or on subendothelium, in particular fibrinogen, fibrin, fibronectin and collagen [58–61]. This molecule could therefore contribute to the stabilization and surface anchoring of platelet aggregates. Formation of a macromolecular complex between thrombospondin, fibrinogen and GP IIb-IIIa has been proposed as an important step leading to the irreversible aggregation of platelets, while antibodies against thrombospondin have been shown to partially inhibit aggregation in response to ADP, thrombin and collagen [62]. A further component of platelet α-granules, the integral membrane glycoprotein GMP–140 (granule membrane protein 140), may also be involved in long term stabilization of surface aggregates [63].

Role of thrombin

Since thrombin is detectable within 45 seconds after injury of a blood vessel [64], the role of this enzyme in platelet activation and mobilization of GP IIb-IIIa receptors is of prime importance for the adhesive interactions of platelets in haemostatic and thrombotic processes. Thrombin generation through blood contact with artificial surfaces enhances platelet accumulation on these surfaces [65], while in studies of platelet deposition on Dacron grafts thrombin was found to be the principal mediator of acute high flow platelet dependent graft occlusion [66]. The platelet thrombin receptor has recently been identified by expression cloning and sequencing of its cDNA [67]. This high affinity recognition domain consists of a single polypeptide chain with seven membrane spanning segments and an extracellular amino terminus containing a thrombin sensitive site between arg^{41} and ser^{42}. Cleavage by thrombin creates a new amino terminus which behaves as a tethered ligand, platelet activation being triggered by the interaction of this new amino segment with another region of the receptor. Peptide analogues of this sequence induce similar activation [68]. These recent findings elucidating the mechanism of thrombin interaction with platelets should prove of value for the design of new antithrombotic agents, in particular synthetic peptide inhibitors of thrombin activity [66].

Conclusions

Platelet adhesion is the first event in the haemostatic process and likewise in the formation of pathological thrombi. Adhesion depends on haemodynamic factors which control platelet transport to the vessel wall and the shear forces acting in the vicinity of the wall and on the interaction of platelet membrane receptors with adhesive proteins present on subendothelium or artificial surfaces or in plasma or platelet α-granules. At high wall shear rates ($> 500\ s^{-1}$), the binding of subendothelial vWF to its receptor GP Ib plays a predominant role. Adhesive interactions involving other components of subendothelium, in particular collagen and fibronectin, become increasingly important at moderate and low shear rates, while adhesion to fibrinogen coated and fibrin surfaces contributes to thrombus formation on artificial vascular implants and to the growth of platelet-fibrin thrombi. Surface spreading and aggregation of platelets are largely mediated by activated GP IIb-IIIa receptors, which interact with a number of adhesive proteins including fibrinogen, vWF and fibronectin. Thrombin plays a key role in platelet activation and in the conversion of fibrinogen to polymerized fibrin incorporated into surface bound aggregates. A greater insight into the mechanisms controlling platelet adhesion to surfaces should enable the development of new antithrombotic drugs, synthetic peptides and monoclonal antibodies directed against specific functional domains of platelet membrane receptors or adhesive proteins.

References

1. Packham, M.A. and Mustard, J.F., "Platelet adhesion", *Prog. Hemostas. Thromb.* 1984, 7: 211–288.
2. Salzman, E.W. and Merrill, E.W., "Interaction of blood with artificial surfaces", in: *Hemostasis and Thrombosis, Basic Principles and Clinical Practice*, (2nd ed.) Col-

man, R.W., Hirsh, J., Marder, V.J. and Salzman, E.W. (Eds). J.B. Lippincott Company, Philadelphia, 1987, 1335–1347.

3. Cazenave, J.-P., "Interaction of platelets with surfaces", in: *Blood-Surface Interactions: Biological Principles Underlying Haemocompatibility with Artificial Materials*, Cazenave, J.-P., Davies, J.A., Kazatchkine, M. D. and van Aken, W.G. (Eds). Elsevier, Amsterdam, 1986, 89–105.
4. Hawiger, J., "Platelet-vessel wall interactions: platelet adhesion and aggregation", *Atherosclerosis Reviews* 1990, 21: 165–186.
5. Baumgartner, H.R. and Haudenschildt, C., "Adhesion of blood platelets to subendothelium", *Ann. NY Acad. Sci.* 1972, 201: 22–36.
6. Sakariassen, K.S., Aarts, P.A.M.M., de Groot, P.G., Houdijk, W.P.M. and Sixma, J.J., "A perfusion chamber to investigate platelet interaction in flowing blood with human vessel wall cells, their extracellular matrix and purified components", *J. Lab. Clin. Med.* 1983, 102: 522–535.
7. Adams, G.A. and Feuerstein, I.A., "Kinetics of platelet adhesion and aggregation on protein-coated surfaces: morphology and release from dense granules", *ASAIO J.* 1981, 4: 90–99.
8. Mulvihill, J.N., Huisman, H.G., Cazenave, J.-P., van Mourik, J.A. and van Aken, W.G., "The use of monoclonal antibodies to human platelet membrane glycoprotein IIb-IIIa to quantitate platelet deposition on artificial surfaces", *Thromb. Haemostas.* 1987, 58: 724–731.
9. Aarts, P.A.M.M., Bolhuis, P.A., Sakariassen, K.S., Heethaar, R.M. and Sixma, J.J., "Red blood cell size is important for adherence of blood platelets to artery subendothelium", *Blood* 1983, 62: 214–220.
10. Turitto, V.T. and Weiss, H.J., "Rheological factors influencing platelet interaction with vessel surfaces", *Journal of Rheology* 1979, 23: 735–749.
11. de Groot, P.G. and Sixma, J.J., "Platelet adhesion", *Brit. J. Haematol.* 1990, 75: 308–312.
12. Wagner, D.D., Olmsted, J.B. and Marder, V.J., "Immunolocalization of von Willebrand protein in Weibel-Palade bodies of human endothelial cells", *J. Cell Biol.* 1982, 95: 355–360.
13. Hoyer, L.W., "The factor VIII complex: structure and function", *Blood* 1981, 58: 1–13.
14. Lopez-Fernandez, M.F., Ginsberg, M.H., Ruggeri, Z.M., Batille, F.J. and Zimmerman, T.S., "Multimeric structure of platelet factor VIII / von Willebrand factor: the presence of larger multimers and their reassociation with thrombin-stimulated platelets", *Blood* 1982, 60: 1132–1138.
15. Lopez, J.A., Chung, D.W., Fujikawa, K., Hagen, F.S., Papayannopoulou, T. and Roth, G.J., "Cloning of the α chain of human platelet glycoprotein Ib: a transmembrane protein with homology to leucine-rich-α_2-glycoprotein", *Proc. Natl. Acad. Sci. USA* 1987, 84: 5615–5619.
16. Mohri, H., Fujimura, Y., Shima, M., Yoshioka, A., Houghten, R.A., Ruggeri, Z.M. and Zimmerman, T.S., "Structure of the von Willebrand domain interacting with glycoprotein Ib", *J. Biol. Chem.* 1988, 263: 17901–17904.
17. Roth, G.J., "Developing relationships: arterial platelet adhesion, glycoprotein Ib, and leucine-rich glycoproteins", *Blood* 1991, 77: 5–19.
18. Weiss, H.J., Turitto, V.T. and Baumgartner, H.R., "Effect of shear rate on platelet interaction with subendothelium in citrated and native blood: I. Shear rate-dependent decrease of adhesion in Bernard-Soulier syndrome", *J. Lab. Clin. Med.* 1978, 92: 750.
19. Tschopp, T.B., Weiss, H.J. and Baumgartner, H.R., "Decreased adhesion of platelets to subendothelium in von Willebrand's disease", *J. Lab. Clin. Med.* 1974, 83: 296.
20. Ruan, C., Tobelem, G., McMichael, A.J., Drouet, L., Legrand, Y., Degos, L., Kieffer, N., Lee, H. and Caen, J.P., "Monoclonal antibody to human platelet glycoprotein I", *Brit. J. Haematol.* 1981, 49: 511.
21. Sixma, J.J., Sakariassen, K.S., Stel, H.V., Houdijk, W. P.M., In den Maur, D.W., Hamer, R.J., de Groot, P.G. and van Mourik, J.A., "Functional domains on von Willebrand

factor. Recognition of discrete tryptic fragments by monoclonal antibodies that inhibit interaction of von Willebrand factor with platelets and with collagen", *J. Clin. Invest.* 1984, 74: 736.

22. Weiss, H.J., Turitto, V.T. and Baumgartner, H.R., "Platelet adhesion and thrombus formation on subendothelium in platelets deficient in glycoproteins IIb-IIIa and storage organelles", *Blood* 1986, 67: 322–331.
23. Piotrowicz, R.S., Orchekowski, R.P., Nugent, D.J., Yameda, K.Y. and Kunicki, T.J., "Glycoprotein Ic-IIa functions as an activation-independent fibronectin receptor on human platelets", *J. Cell Biol.* 1988, 106: 1359–13564.
24. Plow, E.F., McEver, R.P., Coller, B.S., Woods, V.L. Jr., Marguerie, G.A. and Ginsberg, M.H., "Related binding mechanisms for fibrinogen, fibronectin, von Willebrand factor and thrombospondin on thrombin-stimulated human platelets", *Blood* 1985, 66: 724–727.
25. Barnes, D.W., Silnutzer, J., See, C. and Shaffer, M., "Characterization of human serum spreading factor with monoclonal antibody", *Proc. Natl. Acad. Sci. USA* 1983, 80: 1362–1366.
26. Staatz, W.D., Rajpara, S.M., Wayner, E.A., Carter, W.G. and Santoro, S.A., "The membrane glycoprotein Ia-IIa (VLA–2) complex mediates the Mg^{++}-dependent adhesion of platelets to collagen", *J. Cell Biol.* 1989, 108: 1917–1924.
27. Nieuwenhuis, H.K., Akkerman, J.W.N., Houdijk, W.P.M. and Sixma, J.J., "Human blood platelets showing no response to collagen fail to express surface glycoprotein Ia", *Nature* 1985, 318: 470–472.
28. Nieuwenhuis, H.K., Sakariassen, K.S., Houdijk, W.P. M., Nievelstein, P.F.E.M. and Sixma, J.J., "Deficiency of platelet membrane glycoprotein Ia associated with a decreased platelet adhesion to subendothelium: a defect in platelet spreading", *Blood* 1986, 68: 692–695.
29. Staatz, W.D., Fok, K.F., Zutter, M.M., Adams, S.P., Rodriguez, B.A. and Santoro, S.A., "Identification of a tetrapeptide recognition sequence for the $\alpha_2\beta_1$ integrin in collagen", *J. Biol. Chem.* 1991, 266: 7363–7367.
30. Santoro, S.A., Walsh, J.J., Staatz, W.D. and Baranski, K.J., "Distinct determinants on collagen support $\alpha_2\beta_1$ integrin-mediated platelet adhesion and platelet activation", *Cell Regulation* 1991, 2: 905–913.
31. Houdijk, W.P.M., Sakariassen, K.S. and Sixma, J.J., "Role of factor VIII-von Willebrand factor and fibronectin in the interaction of platelets in flowing blood with monomeric and fibrillar collagen types I and III", *J. Clin. Invest.* 1985, 75: 531–540.
32. Ill, C.R., Engvall, E. and Ruoslahti, E., "Adhesion of platelets to laminin in the absence of activation", *J. Cell Biol.* 1984, 99: 2140–2145.
33. Sonnenberg, A., Modderman, P.W. and Hogervorst, F., "Laminin receptor on platelets is the integrin VLA–6", *Nature* 1988, 336: 487–489.
34. Ordinas, A., Diaz-Ricart, M., Bastida, E., Escolar, G., Castillo, R., Tandon, N.N. and Jamieson, G.A., "The role of subendothelial laminin and platelet laminin receptors in haemostasis", *Nouv. Rev. Fr. Hematol.* 1992, 34: 61–65.
35. Legrand, Y.J. and Fauvel-Lafève, F., "Molecular mechanism of the interaction of subendothelial microfibrils with blood platelets", *Nouv. Rev. Fr. Hematol.* 1992, 34: 17–25.
36. Packham, M.A., Evans, G., Glynn, M.F. and Mustard, J.F., "The effect of plasma proteins on the interaction of platelets with glass surfaces", *J. Lab. Clin. Med.* 1969, 73: 686–697.
37. Zucker, M.B. and Vroman, L., "Platelet adhesion induced by fibrinogen adsorbed to glass", *Proc. Soc. Exp. Biol. Med.* 1969, 131: 318–320.
38. Mosher, D.F., "Influence of proteins on platelet-surface interactions", in: *Interaction of the Blood with Natural and Artificial Surfaces*, Salzman, E.W. (Ed). Marcel Dekker, New York, 1981, 85–101.
39. Brash, J.L., "Protein adsorption at the solid-solution interface in relation to blood-material interactions", in: *Proteins at Interfaces: Physicochemical and Biochemical Studies*, Brash, J.L. and Horbett, T.A. (Eds). ACS Symposium Series, American Chemical Society, Washington DC, 1987, 490–506.

40. Doolittle, R.F., "Fibrinogen and fibrin", *Annu. Rev. Biochem.* 1984, 53: 195–229.
41. Hawiger, J., Timmons, S., Kloczewiak, M., Strong, D.D. and Doolittle, R.F., "Gamma and alpha chains of human fibrinogen possess sites reactive with human platelet receptors", *Proc. Natl. Acad. Sci. USA* 1982, 79: 2068–2071.
42. Ruoshlati, E. and Pierschbacher, M.D., "New perspectives in cell adhesion: RGD and integrins", *Science* 1987, 238: 491–497.
43. Pidard, D., "The platelet fibrinogen receptor: a model for analysis of the mechanisms of cellular adhesion and their modifications in pathology", *Path. Biol.* 1989, 37: 1107–1113.
44. Coller, B.S., Peerschke, E.I., Scuder, L.E. and Sullivan, C.A., "A murine monoclonal antibody that completely blocks the binding of fibrinogen to platelets produces a thrombasthenic-like state in normal platelets and binds glycoproteins IIb and/or IIIa", *J. Clin. Invest.* 1983, 72: 325–338.
45. Nachman, R.L. and Leung, L.L.K., "Complex formation of platelet membrane glycoproteins IIb and IIIa with fibrinogen", *J. Clin. Invest.* 1982, 69: 263–269.
46. Clemetson, K.J. and Luscher, E.F., "Membrane glycoprotein abnormalities in pathological platelets", *Biochim. Biophys. Acta* 1988, 947: 53–73.
47. Ruggeri, Z.M., Bader, R. and DeMarco, L., "Glanzmann's thrombasthenia: deficient binding of von Willebrand factor to thrombin-stimulated platelets", *Proc. Natl. Acad. Sci. USA* 1982, 79: 6038–6041.
48. Ginsberg, M.H., Forsyth, J., Lightsey, A., Chediak, J. and Plow, E.F., "Reduced surface expression and binding of fibronectin by thrombin-stimulated thrombasthenic platelets", *J. Clin. Invest.* 1983, 71: 1–8.
49. Thiagarajan, P. and Kelly, K.L., "Exposure of binding sites for vitronectin on platelets following stimulation", *J. Biol. Chem.* 1988, 263: 3035–3038.
50. Yasuda, T., Gold, H.K. and Fallon, J.T., "Monoclonal antibody against the platelet glycoprotein (GP) IIb/IIIa receptor prevents coronary artery reocclusion after reperfusion with recombinant tissue-type plasminogen activator in dogs", *J. Clin. Invest.* 1988, 81: 1284–1291.
51. Hanson, S.R., Pareti, F.I. and Ruggeri, Z.M., "Effects of monoclonal antibodies against the platelet glycoprotein IIb/IIIa complex on thrombosis and hemostasis in the baboon", *J. Clin. Invest.* 1988, 81: 149–158.
52. Kloczewiak, M., Timmons, S., Bednarek, M.A., Sakon, M. and Hawiger, J., "Platelet receptor recognition domain on the gamma chain of human fibrinogen and its synthetic peptide analogs", *Biochemistry* 1989, 28: 2915–2919.
53. Cook, J.C., Huang, T.-F., Rucinski, B., Tuma, R.F., Williams, J.A. and Niewiarowski, S., "Inhibition of platelet hemostatic plug formation by trigramin, a novel RGD containing peptide", *Circulation* 1988, 78: II–313.
54. Shiba, E., Lindon, J. and Kushner, L., "Changes in conformation of fibrinogen adsorbed on polymer surfaces detected by polyclonal and monoclonal antibodies", *Circulation* 1988, 78: II–622.
55. Isenberg, W.M., McEver, R.P., Phillips, D.R. and Shuman, M.A., "The platelet fibrinogen receptor: an immunogold-surface replica study of agonist-induced ligand binding and receptor clustering", *J. Cell Biol.* 1987, 104: 1655–1663.
56. Jen, C.J. and Lin, J.S., "Direct observation of platelet adhesion to fibrinogen- and fibrin-coated surfaces", *Amer. J. Physiol.* 1991, 261: H1457–1463.
57. Lawler, J.W., Slayter, H.S. and Coligan, J.E., "Isolation and characterization of a high molecular weight glycoprotein from human blood platelets", *J. Biol. Chem.* 1978, 253: 8609–8616.
58. Leung, L.L.K. and Nachman, R.L., "Complex formation of platelet thrombospondin with fibrinogen", *J. Clin. Invest.* 1982, 70: 542–549.
59. Bale, M.D., Westrick, L.G. and Mosher, D.F., "Incorporation of thrombospondin into fibrin clots", *J. Biol. Chem.* 1985, 260: 7502–7508.
60. Lahav, J., Schwartz, M.A. and Hynes, R.O., "Analysis of platelet adhesion with a radioactive chemical cross-linking reagent: interaction of thrombospondin with fibronectin

and collagen", *Cell* 1982, 31: 253–262.

61. Galvin, N.J., Vance, P.M., Dixit, V.M., Fink, B. and Frazier, W.A., "Interaction of human thrombospondin with types I-V collagen: direct binding and electron microscopy", *J. Cell Biol.* 1987, 104: 1413–1422.
62. Parmentier, S., Kaplan, C., Catimel, B. and McGregor, J.L., "New families of adhesion molecules play a vital role in platelet functions", *Immunology Today* 1990, 11: 225–227.
63. Johnston, G.I., Cook, R.G. and McEver, R.P., "Cloning of GMP–140, granule membrane protein, of platelets and endothelium: sequence similarities to proteins involved in cell adhesion and inflammation", *Cell* 1989, 56: 1033–1044.
64. Teitel, J.M., Bauer, K.A., Lau, H.J. and Rosenberg, R.D., "Studies of the prothrombin activation pathway utilizing radioimmunoassays for the F_2/F_{1+2} fragment and thrombin-antithrombin complex", *Blood* 1982, 59: 1086–1097.
65. Mulvihill, J.N., Davies, J.A., Toti, F., Freyssinet, J.-M. and Cazenave, J.-P., "Thrombin stimulated platelet accumulation on protein coated glass capillaries: role of adhesive platelet α-granule proteins", *Thromb. Haemostas.* 1989, 62: 989–995.
66. Hanson, S.R. and Harker, L.A., "Interruption of acute platelet-dependent thrombosis by the synthetic antithrombin D-phenylalanyl-L-prolyl-L-arginyl-chloromethyl ketone", *Proc. Natl. Acad. Sci. USA* 1988, 85: 3184–3188.
67. Vu, T.-K., Hung, D.T., Wheaton, V.I. and Coughlin, S.R., "Molecular cloning of a functional thrombin receptor reveals a novel proteolytic mechanism of receptor activation", *Cell* 1991, 64: 1057–1068.
68. Vassallo, R.R. Jr., Kieber-Emmons, T., Cichowski, K. and Brass, L.F., "Structure-function relationships in the activation of platelet thrombin receptors by receptor-derived peptides", *J. Biol. Chem.* 1992, 267: 6081–6085.

7. Role of thrombin in platelet-biomaterial interactions

S. R. HANSON
Associate Professor of Medicine, Emory University School of Medicine, Atlanta, Georgia, USA

Introduction

Since no artificial surface is completely inert towards blood, thrombosis and thromboembolism complicate to some extent the use of all blood-contacting cardiovascular devices, whether intended for short-term or long-term applications [1]. Anticoagulant therapy is generally required to maintain device function with acceptable or low risk, implying an important role for the procoagulant enzyme thrombin in the thrombotic process. When devices are placed in the arterial circulation, the accumulation of blood platelets serves to localize and accelerate coagulation reactions leading to the formation of thrombus which may be composed almost entirely of platelets. These platelet masses may subsequently impair device function, or embolize to produce ischemia in distal microcirculatory beds. Platelet-biomaterial interactions have generally been resistant to conventional anticoagulant therapy (e.g., heparin), suggesting either that heparin is limited in its ability to affect this process, or that other thrombin-independent pathways of platelet recruitment may be of relatively greater importance [1, 2]. However, recent studies with more potent and specific inhibitors of the thrombin-platelet interaction have suggested that thrombin is indeed a key physiologic agonist for platelet activation *in vivo*. These observations are discussed below.

In addition to its actions on platelets, thrombin mediates several other important reactions in hemostasis, including conversion of fibrinogen to fibrin with cleavage fibrinopeptides A and B, and activation of coagulation Factor V, Factor VIII, and Factor XIII [3]. Thrombin may also act as an anticoagulant enzyme since, following binding to endothelial cell thrombomodulin, thrombin cannot activate platelets but rather activates protein C which inhibits coagulation by inactivating Factors Va and VIIIa [3–5]. Cell membrane phospholipids accelerate two critical steps leading to the production of thrombin: Factor X activation and the conversion of prothrombin to thrombin. *In vivo*, these reactions may proceed efficiently only in the presence of catalytic platelet phospholipids, which thus serve to localize the clotting reactions leading to the generation of thrombin [5]. In blood, thrombin is primarily inhibited by antithrombin III, a reaction that is potently catalyzed by heparin. While

Y. F. Missirlis and J.-L. Wautier (eds.), The Role of Platelets in Blood-Biomaterial Interactions, 81–93.

thrombin binding to fibrinogen *substrate* sites leads to fibrinogen cleavage and release of fibrinopeptides, the binding of thrombin's exosite domain to *non-substrate* sites on fibrin may serve to localize thrombin activity, preserve its catalytic potential, and prevent its inactivation by heparin-antithrombin III [6, 7].

Thrombin can effect responses from a variety of cell types including endothelial cells, smooth muscle cells, fibroblasts, and platelets, and is also chemotactic for monocytes [8]. Platelet responses include the release of alpha granule and dense granule contents, expression of the glycoprotein (GP) IIb/IIIa receptor for fibrinogen and other adhesive molecules, and formation platelet aggregates and thrombi. While these responses may be elicited by a variety of agonists including adenosine diphosphate (ADP), epinephrine, collagen, and calcium ionophores, thrombin is considered to be the physiologic agonist [9]. Interestingly, individual platelets may be quite heterogeneous in their capacity to secrete granular contents in response to thrombin [10]. In general, the cellular responses to thrombin are thought to be mediated through cell surface receptors coupled via G proteins to intracellular enzymes such as phospholipase C which generate second messengers that mediate platelet activation. For example, platelet stimulation by thrombin may result in tyrosine phosphorylation, an increase in cytosolic Ca^{++}, and inhibition of cyclic adenosine monophosphate (cAMP) formation [11–13]. While a potential role for thrombin in these platelet-associated events has been recognized for some time, the mechanisms by which thrombin causes platelet activation, and the identity of the platelet receptor(s) which regulate this process, have been controversial [9]. However, a major advance in our understanding was achieved with the recent cloning of a functional thrombin receptor [13]. Insights derived from these studies, which are important for understanding the role of thrombin in platelet-biomaterial interactions, will be reviewed briefly.

Thrombin-platelet interactions

Early attempts to identify thrombin receptor sites on platelets involved measurement of kinetic parameters in traditional ligand-platelet binding studies, and assessment of hydrolysis of specific platelet membrane glycoproteins [9]. Initial interest focused on GP Ib, the platelet receptor for von Willebrand factor which mediates platelet adhesion to collagen and perhaps other subendothelial vessel wall components [9, 14]. GP Ib is relatively abundant on the platelet surface ($\sim$ 15,000 copies per platelet), and thrombin has been observed to bind to both solubilized and membrane-associated GP Ib, as well as to the large extracellular domain portion of GP Ib, glycocalicin. Thrombin binding is deficient with platelets from patients with Bernard-Soulier disease, which lack GP Ib. However, GP Ib is not cleaved by thrombin, but rather inhibits thrombin's proteolytic activity. Further, GP Ib binds catalytically inactive thrombin which cannot activate platelets. Thus while it is unlikely that

GP Ib is a functional thrombin receptor, it may serve as an ancillary binding site for localizing thrombin at the platelet surface. Glycoprotein V has also been proposed as a receptor/substrate involved in platelet activation since it is the only known platelet membrane protein that is hydrolyzed by thrombin, with release of a large (M_r = 69,000) fragment [9, 14]. However, hydrolysis of GP V does not correlate with platelet activation, which is also unaffected by antibodies against GP V. These results argue against GP V as a functional thrombin receptor.

The most important recent development in this area has been the cloning and characterization of a functional thrombin receptor by Vu, *et al.* [13]. Because of difficulties with classical binding studies, these investigators adopted an approach whereby the cDNA encoding a functional thrombin receptor was isolated by direct expression cloning in *Xenopus* oocytes. Oocytes transfected with the receptor responded to thrombin (in terms of Ca^{++} release), but did not respond to catalytically inactive thrombin, or to thrombin in the presence of hirugen (the carboxy-terminal dodecapeptide from the leech-derived antithrombin hirudin) which specifically inhibits thrombin's anion binding exosite without affecting catalytic site function. These responses mimicked those seen with intact platelets. The deduced amino sequence revealed structural similarities with the large family of seven transmembrane "G-protein coupled" receptors. However, identification of a functional thrombin receptor revealed a novel mechanism of receptor activation, which is illustrated in Figure 1. In this model, the thrombin receptor's relatively long (100 residue) extracellular tail is cleaved between arginine 41 and serine 42, exposing a new amino terminal sequence which functions as a tethered ligand peptide for the receptor. Studies in support of this model demonstrated that oocytes expressing mutant thrombin receptors lacking the arginine cleavage site failed to respond to thrombin, while peptides mimicking the new amino terminus, which contains the sequence SFLLRN (Ser-Phe-Leu-Leu-Arg-Asn), fully activated both the receptor expressed in oocytes as well as intact platelets [13]. Platelet stimulation by the SFLLRN sequence was subsequently shown to account fully for several features of the platelet response to thrombin, thereby implicating thrombin's proteolytic activity for its receptor and the formation of a tethered ligand [11–13]. Other recent studies supporting this model have shown that: (1) replacing the thrombin receptor cleavage site with that for another enzyme (enterokinase) completely switched the receptor's specificity [15], (2) the thrombin receptor's hirudin-like sequence can bind to thrombin's anion-binding exosite [16], and (3) polyclonal antibodies to the hirudin-like domain in the receptor's extracellular tail block thrombin-induced platelet aggregation [17]. These studies indicate that the cloned thrombin receptor, and its cleavage to expose the tethered ligand peptide, are necessary for thrombin-induced platelet activation [18].

These studies raise a number of interesting questions. Do different thrombin receptor subtypes exist, perhaps on different cell types? What are the intracellular signalling mechanisms mediated by the thrombin receptor? Do

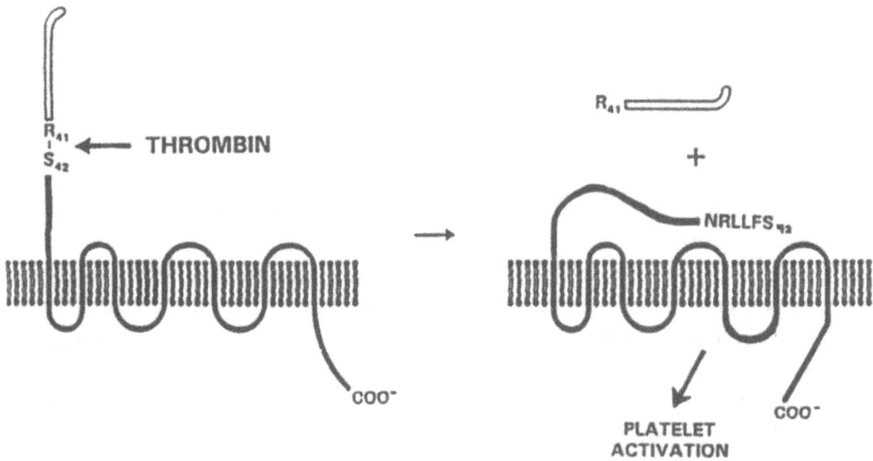

Figure 1. Thrombin receptor activation. Cleavage of the thrombin receptor between Arg (41) and Ser (42) yields a new amino terminal peptide having the sequence SFLLRN which acts as a tethered ligand to activate the receptor. (Adapted from Vu *et al.*, *Cell* 1991, 64: 1065).

other platelet membrane glycoproteins, such as GP Ib, play a role by locally concentrating or inhibiting thrombin? Binding studies using monoclonal antibodies have indicated that the thrombin receptor on platelets is present in relatively low copy number (~ 1,000 receptors per platelet). How many receptors must be cleaved, and in what temporal sequence, before a platelet becomes activated? Do activated platelets circulate? What are the mechanisms of receptor desensitization following cleavage by thrombin or activation by peptide agonists? Does the tethered peptide undergo additional cleavages which inactivate the receptor, as has been suggested [19]? Are other platelet activating factors such as ADP or thromboxane A_2 cooperative in thrombin-induced platelet activation? To what extent are these reactions governed by local conditions of blood flow, shear rate, and device geometry? What are the prospects for effective inhibition of *in vivo* thrombus formation by targeting the thrombin receptor, e.g., by using monoclonal antibody or synthetic peptide antagonists? Since these issues are being actively addressed in a number of laboratories, it is anticipated that future work will substantially further our understanding of basic mechanisms and perhaps lead to development of novel therapeutic strategies.

Role of thrombin in platelet-biomaterial interactions

Initial platelet-surface reactions

When artificial surfaces contact blood they first acquire a layer of plasma proteins through dynamic processes of competitive adsorption/desorption. Like other plasma proteins, prothrombin can adsorb to surfaces such as polyethylene [20], raising the possibility that certain surfaces could locally concentrate prothrombin relative to plasma levels. Following conversion of prothrombin by prothrombinase complex, thrombin derived from the adsorbed protein layer could participate in the activation and accumulation of blood platelets, or formation of fibrin. In general, relationships between material surface properties, protein adsorption, and subsequent platelet-surface interactions are poorly understood since many plasma proteins may interact with surfaces in a complex manner that changes with time, and which may be also influenced by the subsequent surface interactions of platelets and other blood cells.

The earliest event following blood-surface contact which can be identified morphologically is the adhesion of blood platelets. Since thrombin is presumably unavailable at this time, initial platelet attachment is thought to be mediated through the platelet GP Ib and GP IIb/IIIa membrane receptors for fibrinogen and other adhesive glycoproteins. Thus while the adhesion of platelets to subendothelial tissue components is thought to depend on the binding of von Willebrand factor to GP Ib, initial platelet attachment to polyethylene and microvascular ePTFE (expanded polytetrafluoroethylene) vascular grafts requires GP IIb/IIIa, although GP Ib is required for the accumulation of subsequent platelet layers and may influence the adhesion process as well [21, 22].

Following initial platelet attachment, platelet activation and aggregate formation result in the expression of platelet membrane phospholipids which potently accelerate the conversion of Factor X to Factor Xa (tenase complex) and the conversion of prothrombin to thrombin (prothrombinase complex). Localized thrombin generation at the platelet surface thus initates a positive feedback mechanism whereby thrombin produces further activation of platelets and their recruitment into the growing aggregate. This process is limited by a number of factors, including the inhibitory effects of antithrombin III and activated protein C, thrombin binding to fibrin, rapid dilution of procoagulant materials under blood flow, and the local depletion or consumption of platelets and perhaps other factors at sites of aggregate growth. With the formation of thrombi which perturb the blood flow field, relationships between platelets, surfaces, and prothrombotic factors become complex. Under low flow conditions, the focal generation of procoagulant material may cause distal propagation of thrombus, as in venous thrombosis, which depends on thrombin activity and may be inhibited by anticoagulants such as heparin. Under other conditions, upstream thrombus growth may impair downstream thrombus formation, presumably due to depletion of the fluid boundary layer of platelets and clotting factors [23]. In general, the fluid mechanics of thrombus formation (and thrombin generation) in flowing whole blood systems, and its dependence on blood exposure time, hematologic variables, and the nature of the initiating substrate surface, is poorly understood. Interestingly, theoretical analyses of concentration profiles of platelet-activating agents near growing thrombi have predicted that levels of released ADP and thromboxane A_2 may be marginally large enough to cause platelet activation, while levels of locally generated thrombin may be much greater than required for platelet stimulation [24, 25]. The prediction of a central role for thrombin is also in accord with results obtained in experimental *in vivo* thrombosis models, as discussed below.

Platelet thrombus formation in vivo

Studies with newer antithrombotic agents which directly inhibit thrombin's catalytic activity have provided convincing evidence for a critical role of thrombin in animal models of arterial thrombosis [26, 27]. Since these agents inhibit all thrombin catalytic site functions, including activation of protein C and cleavage of fibrinogen, the role of thrombin's action on platelets alone, while undoubtedly important, is difficult to assess unambiguously. In addition, most models have focused on the response to vascular injury, rather than mechanisms of thrombus formation associated with artificial materials and prosthetic devices.

To address these issues we have employed a baboon arteriovenous (AV) shunt model of thrombus formation as illustrated in Figure 2. In this system a chronic AV shunt composed of nonthrombogenic silicone rubber tubing is established between the femoral artery and vein. Between proximal and distal shunt segments are interposed various artificial surfaces which can include smooth-walled tubings, textured materials such as vascular grafts (i.e., a Dacron graft as in Figure 2), or clinical devices such as hemodialyzers and endovascular stents [28]. In comparison with other animal models and *ex vivio* test systems, this approach has several advantages: (1) the hemostatic system of the baboon resembles closely that of man, (2) device geometry and blood flow parameters are readily controlled and measured, and (3) blood-material interactions may be studied both short-term or long-term, in the presence or absence of anticoagulants [28]. In addition, since surfaces or devices are interposed between segments of essentially nonreactive polymeric tubing, platelet deposition and thrombus formation are initiated through mechanisms that depend on the physicochemical properties of the materials being tested, rather than on tissue factor initiation of the extrinsic coagulation mechanism [3] that occurs upon vessel injury (e.g, with placement of indwelling catheters or construction of surgical graft anastomoses). Platelet thrombus formation is assessed by dynamic and noninvasive gamma scintillation imaging of platelets labelled with ^{111}Indium, and by gamma counting of ^{125}Iodine-labeled fibrinogen. These models have been described in detail [28, 29].

To assess the role of thrombin's enzymatic activity on platelet thrombus formation we initially studied the synthetic peptide antithrombin D-Phe-Pro-Arg chloromethylketone (PPACK) which irreversibly inactivates thrombin by forming a covalent bond at thrombin's catalytic site [29]. The model employed was that of Figure 2, where a segment of knitted Dacron vas-

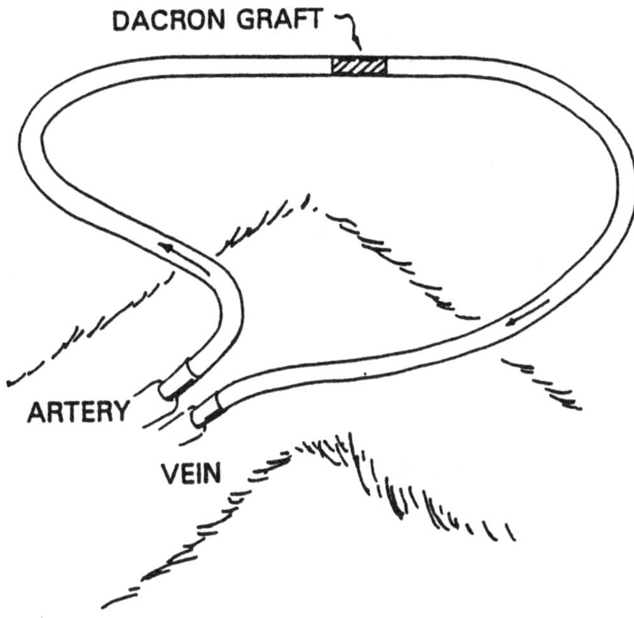

Figure 2. Arteriovenous shunt model for evaluating blood responses to biomaterials. Following placement of nonthrombogenic silicone rubber shunts between the femoral artery and vein of normal baboons, test materials or devices (e.g., a Dacron graft) are interposed between proximal and distal shunt segments.

cular graft (4.0 mm i.d.) was exposed to arterial blood flow (100 ml/min) in animals given intravenous PPACK at a dose of 100 nmol/kg-min [29]. The results of this study, given in Figure 3, showed that PPACK virtually abolished platelet deposition (by > 95% after 60 min of graft blood exposure) relative to results obtained in untreated control animals, thus documenting the central role of thrombin in platelet thrombus formation associated with this biomaterial. This study also revealed several other interesting features. First, in the interval between 10–30 min of blood exposure a transient increase in platelet accumulation was observed (Figure 3) suggesting a small thrombin-independent (perhaps GP IIb/IIIa mediated) process in the early formation of platelet aggregates which were, however, unstable over time and lost from the surface through embolization and/or lytic mechanisms. Second, heparin anticoagulation in conventional doses (100 units/kg) did not reduce thrombus formation [29], and even the very high dose of 1,000 units/kg (Figure 3) was only marginally effective. Heparin was also shown to be ineffective for reducing elevated rates of steady-state platelet consumption by chronic shunts composed of various polyurethanes and acrylic hydrogel polymers [30]. These results are now explained by observations that: (1) thrombin bound to fibrin, and Factor Xa bound to platelets, are protected from inactivation by the heparin-antithrombin III complex [6, 7], which may also be stearically excluded from penetrating the thrombus, and (2) platelets secrete a heparin-neutralizing protein, platelet factor 4 [31]. Third, we observed that with cessation of the PPACK infusion thrombus formation rapidly occurred, implying that the inherent reactivity of the underlying substrate was not diminished. Therefore, to determine whether locally deposited thrombin was a factor in maintaining the "thrombogenicity" of platelet-rich thrombi, we allowed thrombus to form on Dacron grafts which were then exposed under static flow conditions to high concentrations of PPACK (10 mg/ml). This treatment permanently abolished the capacity of these thrombi to accumulate additional platelets [32], documenting the importance of thrombus-associated thrombin in this process. Finally, it is interesting to speculate why thrombus (and thrombin) forms at all, or so robustly, in this artificial surface model which excludes tissue factor activation of the extrinsic coagulation pathway. It is possible that the intrinsic coagulation pathway may be initiated through surface activation of Factor XII, or through activation of Factor XI by initially adherent platelets [33]. Alternatively, there may always be trace levels of circulating thrombin (or Factor Xa) which can initiate clotting at vulnerable (nonendothelialized) sites. Although these possibilities await clarification, it is clear from these studies that artificial surfaces in the absence of tissue injury can stimulate the rapid production of thrombin which in turn promotes the local accumulation of thrombus.

The importance of the thrombin pathway for platelet deposition onto artificial surfaces, and its susceptability for inhibition, may also depend upon local flow conditions. For example, we have studied in the same primate model complex devices having regions of sudden expansion-contraction which exhibit low shear flow, flow recirculation and stasis [34]. Under these conditions heparin and other antithrombins effectively block platelet deposition, fibrin formation, and thrombus propagation [34]. These results suggest that thrombi formed under low shear conditions, which may be composed largely of fibrin, are generated primarily through the actions of solution-phase thrombin, as opposed to thrombin sequestered in platelet-rich arterial thrombi. Thus heparin is widely used and clinically effective in the treatment of venous thrombosis, and for preventing clot formation in devices having complex flow geometries such as hemodialyzers, oxygenators, and cardiopulmonary bypass apparatus [1]. However, due to the limitations of heparin therapy discussed above, other direct antithrombins could be expected to be more efficacious in these settings as well. For example, when hollow fiber artificial kidneys were studied in primates, PPACK therapy was significantly more effective than heparin in preventing platelet deposition, and for preserving hollow fiber bundle volume and device function [35].

Given the importance of thrombin in platelet-mediated events, there has been considerable recent interest in the development and testing of both natural and synthetic compounds which inhibit either thrombin's activity or its production *in vivo*. A number of these agents, and the coagulation pathways targeted, are shown in Figure 4. Using the model given in Figure 2 with a Dacron artificial surface we have studied several derivatives of PPACK

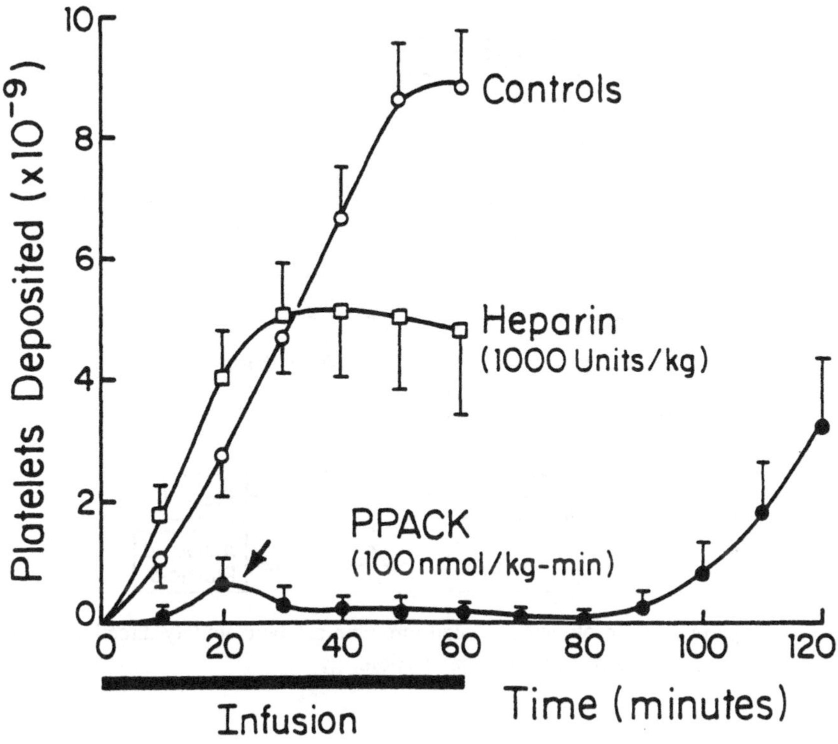

Figure 3. Platelet thrombus formation on Dacron grafts incorporated into arteriovenous shunts in baboons. In animals given the potent antithrombin PPACK, thrombus formation is modest between 10–30 min of blood exposure (arrow), declines until 60 min, and increases rapidly thereafter when the PPACK infusion is discontinued. By comparison, heparin therapy produces only a modest effect. (Adapted from Hanson, S. R., Harker, L. A., *Proc. Natl. Acad. Sci. USA*, 85: 3186).

including the tripeptide (D-FPR), the aldehyde (D-FPRH), and boroarginyl (D-FPRBOH) derivatives [36]. We have also studied the polypeptide hirudin produced by the leech *Hirudo medicinalis* which inactivates thrombin by reversible tight complex formation [37]. All of these inhibitors reduce platelet thrombus formation, further documenting the role of thrombin in this process. However, all direct antithrombins produce an increase in bleeding tendency from a small skin incision (standard template bleeding time), demonstrating the importance of thrombin for mediating platelet aggregation in the microvasculature as well as in larger arteries. Interestingly, the carboxy-terminal dodecapeptide of hirudin ("hirugen") which blocks thrombin's anion binding exosite and could affect thrombin's interaction with its receptor, prevented only venous-type thrombus formation when studied in this model [38].

Agents which have been used to block thrombin production include antistasin, an inhibitor of Factor Xa isolated from the leech *Haementeria offici-*

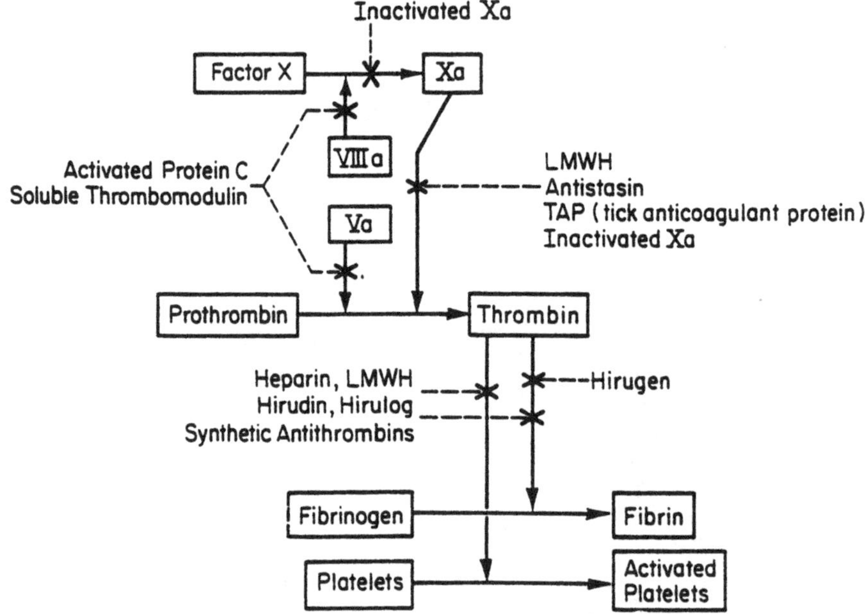

Figure 4. Experimental agents which inhibit thrombin catalytic activity directly, or which block coagulation factors necessary for its production.

nalis, and plasma-derived or recombinant activated protein C (APC) which inactivates the coagulation cofactors Va and VIIIa (Figure 4). These agents also markedly inhibit thrombus formation in the Dacron graft arteriovenous shunt model [39, 40], and interestingly produce less of a bleeding tendency than the direct antithrombins at doses which are comparably antithrombotic. Presumably, under these conditions low levels of thrombin may be formed in the microcirculation via the tissue factor pathway which are adequate for the initial arrest of bleeding. The importance of thrombin-induced activation of protein C pathway for maintaining an anticoagulant state *in vivo* was also shown by infusing thrombin intravenously into baboons [41]. In these studies, thrombin infusion (1–2 units/kg-min) increased circulating APC levels several hundred fold, reduced platelet thrombus formation on Dacron grafts by about 50%, and abolished platelet accumulation in polymeric devices exhibiting low shear flow recirculation and stasis [41]. Thus, paradoxically, while thrombin produced locally at sites of thrombus formation is critical for thrombus growth, systemic thrombin may produce a net antithrombotic effect through activation of the protein C pathway.

Finally, since both the direct and indirect antithrombins discussed above block or prevent all thrombin functions, preliminary studies have been performed targeting the thrombin receptor specifically. When a synthetic peptide antagonist based on the thrombin receptor neoterminal SFLLRN sequence was infused into baboons with Dacron grafts, platelet deposition could be reduced by > 50%, an effect comparable in magnitude to that seen with other antithrombins. Thus these results, if confirmed, imply that platelet aggregate formation *in vivo* occurs predominantly through the action of thrombin on its platelet receptor, rather than in response to other platelet activating factors or through the actions of thrombin on other substrates.

Conclusions

Thrombin is a key agonist for platelet accumulation on artificial surfaces *in vivo*, as shown by the antithrombotic efficacy of agents which inhibit thrombin generation or catalytic activity. These effects may be primarily mediated through the action of thrombin on the platelet thrombin receptor. While many questions remain regarding thrombin receptor signalling and regulation, and the role of local flow conditions, device composition, and geometry, future studies hold considerable promise for understanding surface-platelet-thrombin interactions, and for developing safer and effective therapeutic approaches for the management of cardiovascular device thrombosis.

Acknowledgements

This work was supported by research grants HL 31469 and HL 31950 and RR 00165 from the National Institutes of Health, USA.

References

1. Clagett, G. P., 'Artificial devices in clinical practice', in: *Hemostasis and Thrombosis*, (2nd edition), Colman, R. W., Hirsh, J., Marder, V. J., Salzman, E. W. (Eds). J. B. Lippincott, Philadelphia, PA, 1987, 1348–1366.
2. Cadroy, Y. and Harker, L. A., 'Platelets, thrombosis and antithrombotic therapies', in: *Cardiovascular Pharmacology*, (3rd edition), Antonaccio, M.J. (Ed.), Raven Press, New York, NY, 1990, 515–540.
3. Furie, B. and Furie, B. C., 'Molecular and cellular biology of blood coagulation', *N. Engl. J. Med.* 1992, 326: 800–806.
4. Esmon, N. L., Carroll, R. C., and Esmon, C. T., 'Thrombomodulin blocks the ability of thrombin to activate platelets', *J. Biol. Chem.* 1983, 258: 12238–12242.
5. Mann, K. G., Nesheim, M. E., Church, W. R., Haley, P., and Krishnaswamy, S., 'Surface-dependent reactions of the vitamin K-dependent enzyme complexes', *Blood* 1990, 76: 1–16.
6. Mosesson, M. W., 'Fibrin polymerization and its regulatory role in hemostasis', *J. Lab. Clin. Med.* 1990, 116: 8–17.
7. Weitz, J. I., Hudoba, M., Massel, D., Maraganore, J., and Hirsh, J., 'Clot-bound thrombin is protected from inhibition by, heparin-antithrombin III but is susceptible to inactivation by antithrombin III-independent inhibitors', *J. Clin. Invest.* 1990, 86: 385–391.
8. Shuman, M. A., 'Thrombin-cellular interactions', *Ann. NY Acad. Sci.* 1986, 485: 228–239.

9. Fitzgerald, L. A. and Phillips, D. R., 'Platelet membrane glycoproteins', in: *Hemostasis and Thrombosis*, (2nd edition), Colman, R. W., Hirsh, J., Marder, V. J., Salzman, E. W. (Eds). J. B. Lippincott, Philadelphia, PA, 1987, 572–593.
10. Johnston, G. I., Pickett, E. B., McEver, R. P., and George, J. N., 'Heterogeneity of platelet secretion in response to thrombin demonstrated by fluorescence flow cytometry', *Blood* 1987, 69: 1401–1403.
11. Huang, R., Sorisky, A., Church, W. R., Simons, E. R., and Rittenhouse, S. E., '"Thrombin" receptor-directed ligand accounts for activation by thrombin of platelet phospholipase C and accumulation of 3-phosphorylated phosphoinosotides', *J. Biol. Chem.* 1991, 266: 18435–18438.
12. Vassallo, R. R., Kieber-Emmons, T., Cichowski, K., and Brass, L. F., 'Structure-function relationships in the activation of platelet thrombin receptors by receptor-derived peptides', *J. Biol. Chem.* 1992, 267: 6081–6085.
13. Vu, T. H., Hung, D., Wheaton, V., and Coughlin, S. R., 'Molecular cloning of a functional thrombin receptor reveals a novel proteolytic mechanism of receptor activation', *Cell* 1991, 64: 1057–1068.
14. Kieffer, N. and Phillips, D. R., 'Platelet membrane glycoproteins: Functions in cellular interactions', *Annu. Rev. Cell. Biol.* 1990, 6: 329–357.
15. Vu, T. H., Wheaton, V. I., Hung, D. T., Charo, I., and Coughlin, S. R., 'Domains specifying thrombin-receptor interaction', *Nature* 1991, 353: 674–677.
16. Hung, D. T., Vu, T. H., Wheaton, V. I., Charo, I., Nelken, N. A., Esmon, N., Esmon, C. T., and Coughlin, S. R., '"Mirror image" antagonists of thrombin-induced platelet activation based on thrombin receptor structure', *J. Clin. Invest.* 1992, 89: 444–450.
17. Hung, D. T., Vu, T. H., Wheaton, V. I., Ishii, K., and Coughlin, S. R., 'Cloned thrombin receptor is necessary for thrombin-induced platelet activation', *J. Clin. Invest.* 1992, 89: 1350–1353.
18. Coughlin, S. R., Vu, T. H., Hung, D. T., and Wheaton, V. I., 'Characterization of a functional thrombin receptor. Issues and opportunities', *J. Clin. Invest.* 1992, 89: 351–355.
19. Coller, B. S., Springer, K. T., Scudder, L. E., and Norton, K. J., 'Studies of peptides derived from a platelet thrombin receptor', *Blood* 1991, 78 (Suppl. 1):394a.
20. Slack, S. M., Bohnert, J. L., and Horbett, T. M., 'The effects of surface chemistry and coagulation factors on fibrinogen adsorption from plasma', *Ann. NY Acad. Sci.* 1987, 516: 223–243.
21. Sheppeck, R. A., Bentz, M., Dickson, C., Hribar, S., White, J., Janosky, J., Berceli, S. A., Borovetz, H. S., and Johnson, P. C., 'Examination of the roles of GP Ib and GP IIb/IIIa in platelet deposition on artificial surfaces using clinical antiplatelet agents and monoclonal antibody blockade', *Blood* 1991, 78: 673–680.
22. Johnson, P. C., Sheppeck, R. A., Hribar, S. R., Bentz, M. L., Janosky, J., and Dickson, S., 'Inhibition of platelet retention on artificial micrografts with monoclonal antibodies and a high affinity peptide directed against platelet menmbrane glycoproteins', *Arteriosclerosis and Thrombosis* 1991, 11: 552–560.
23. Sakariassen, K. S., Weiss, H. J., and Baumgartner, H. R., 'Upstream thrombus growth impairs downstrean thrombogenesis in non-anticoagulated blood: Effect of procoagulant artery subendothelium and non-procoagulant collagen', *Thromb. Haemostas.* 1991, 65: 596–600.
24. Folie, B. J. and McIntire, L. V., 'Mathematical analysis of mural thrombogenesis. Concentration profiles of platelet-activating agents and effects of viscous shear flow', *Biophys. J.* 1989, 56: 1121–1141.
25. Hubbell, J. A. and McIntire, L. V., 'Platelet active concentration profiles near growing thrombi', *Biophys. J.* 1986, 50: 937–945.
26. Jang, I. K., Gold, H. K., Ziskind, A. A., Leinbach, R. C., Fallon, J. T., and Collen, D., 'Prevention of platelet-rich arterial thrombosis by selective thrombin inhibition', *Circulation* 1989, 81: 219–225.

27. Fitzgerald, D. J. and FitzGerald, G. A., 'Role of thrombin and thromboxane A_2 in reocclusion following coronary thrombolysis', *Proc. Natl. Acad. Sci. USA* 1989, 86: 7585–7589.
28. Harker, L. A., Kelly, A. B., and Hanson, S. R., 'Experimental arterial thrombosis in non-human primates', *Circulation* 1991, 83 (suppl IV): IV–41–IV–55.
29. Hanson, S. R. and Harker, L. A., 'Interruption of acute platelet-dependent thrombosis by the synthetic antithrombin D-phenylalanyl-L-prolyl-L-arginyl chloromethylketone', *Proc. Natl. Acad. Sci. USA* 1988, 85: 3184–3188.
30. Hanson, S. R., Harker, L. A., Ratner, B. D., and Hoffman, A. S., 'In vivo evaluation of artificial surfaces using a nonhuman primate model of arterial thrombosis', *J. Lab. Clin. Med.* 1980, 95: 289–304.
31. Hirsh, J., 'Heparin', *N. Engl. J. Med.* 1991, 324: 1565–1574.
32. Lumsden, A. B., Kotzé, H. F., Hanson, S. R., and Harker, L. A., 'Brief topical application of synthetic antithrombin prevents vascular graft thrombosis', *Surgical Forum* 1991, 42: 320–321.
33. Walsh, P. N. and Schmaier, A. H., 'Platelet-coagulant protein interactions', in: *Hemostasis and Thrombosis*, (2nd edition), Colman, R. W., Hirsh, J., Marder, V. J., Salzman, E. W. (Eds). J. B. Lippincott, Philadelphia, PA, 1987, 689–709.
34. Cadroy, Y., Horbett, T. A., and Hanson, S. R., 'Discrimination between platelet and coagulation-mediated mechanisms in a model of complex thrombus formation in vivo', *J. Lab. Clin. Med.* 1989, 113: 436–449.
35. Kelly, A. B., Hanson, S. R., Henderson, L. W., and Harker, L. A., 'Prevention of platelet-dependent occlusion of hollow-fiber hemodialyzers by synthetic antithrombin', *J. Lab. Clin. Med.* 1989, 114: 411–418.
36. Kelly, A. B., Hanson, S. R., Knabb, R., Reilly, T. M., and Harker, L. A., 'Relative antithrombotic potencies and hemostatic risks of reversible D-Phe-Pro-Arg (D-FPR) antithrombin derivatives', *Thromb. Haemostas.* 1991, 65(6): 736.
37. Kelly, A. B., Marzec, U. M., Krupski, W., Bass, A., Cadroy, Y., Hanson, S. R., and Harker, L. A., 'Hirudin interruption of heparin-resistant arterial thrombus formation in baboons', *Blood* 1991, 77: 1006–1012.
38. Cadroy, Y., Maraganore, J. M., Hanson, S. R., and Harker, L. A., 'Selective inhibition by a synthetic hirudin peptide of fibrin-dependent thrombosis in baboons', *Proc. Natl. Acad. Sci. USA* 1991, 88: 1177–1181.
39. Gruber, A., Hanson, S. R., Kelly, A. B., Griffin, J. H., Yan, E., Bang, N., and Harker, L. A., 'Recombinant activated protein C (r-apC) inhibition of platelet-dependent thrombosis', *Circulation* 1990, 82: 578–585.
40. Kelly, A. B., White, D., Hanson, S. R., and Harker, L. A., 'Lasting interruption of arterial thrombosis by inhibition of activated factor X', *Blood* 1991, 78(suppl 1): 187a.
41. Gruber, A., Harker, L. A., Griffin, J. G., and Hanson, S. R., 'Inhibition of thrombosis by induced in vivo activation of the protein C pathway', *Blood* 1991, 78(suppl 1): 184a.

8. Polymorphonuclear leukocytes modulate platelet function

C. CERLETTI, V. EVANGELISTA, M. MOLINO, P. PICCARDONI, N. MAUGERI, and G. DE GAETANO

Giulio Bizzozero Laboratory of Platelet and Leukocyte Pharmacology, Istituto di Ricerche Farmacologiche "Mario Negri", "Mario Negri Sud", 66030 Santa Maria Imbaro, Italy

Introduction

After Giulio Bizzozero in 1882 first reported the simultaneous involvement of leukocytes and platelets in thrombus formation [1], the presence of polymorphonuclear leukocytes (PMN) in hemostatic platelet plug and arterial thrombi has been repeatedly observed by microscopy. The general consensus however was that these cells were only playing a passive role in thrombus formation but were likely involved in the subsequent repair process.

More recently, a number of studies has been performed looking for possible interactions between PMN and platelets to better understand their possible importance in the pathogenesis of thrombosis. Results from *in vitro* studies under different experimental conditions indicated that the mutual modulation of platelet and PMN function is extremely complex also due to different methodologic approaches.

The effect of platelets on PMN function has been recently reviewed [2] and will not be the subject of the present review.

We shall focus our attention indeed on the modulatory role of PMN on platelet function. When platelets are stimulated in the presence of PMN, both inhibitory and stimulatory effects on the platelets have been described, suggesting that different *in vitro* experimental systems may reflect different *in vivo* physiopathological situations.

Platelet inhibition induced by PMN

Supernatants of unstimulated PMN incubated at 37° for 30 minutes contained a platelet inhibitory activity which was compatible with thromboxane-synthase inhibition and/or thromboxane receptor antagonism [3]. At the time of this observation (1980) very little was known on the inhibitory effect of PMN on platelet function [4].

The inhibition of platelet activation by PMN has been further investigated

Y. F. Missirlis and J.-L. Wautier (eds.), The Role of Platelets in Blood-Biomaterial Interactions, 95–106.

in the last few years. After Rimele *et al.* [5] described a "neutrophil-derived relaxing factor" with a pharmacological profile similar to that of endothelium-derived relaxing factor/nitric oxide (EDRF/NO), several *in vitro* studies have shown that unstimulated PMN could inhibit platelet activation through a NO-like activity [6–9]. Washed platelets were stimulated with threshold concentrations of specific agonists, in the absence or presence of PMN with a ratio of cell number within the physiologic range. The inhibitory effect of PMN was generally overcome by increasing platelet agonist concentration, and was independent of PMN stimulation. The use of standard indicators of NO-like activity, such as the amplifier superoxide dismutase, the NO scavengers oxyhemoglobin or methylene blue and the NO synthesis blocker N^g monomethyl–2-arginine methyl-ester has provided indirect evidence for platelet inhibition by PMN-derived NO. This interpretation is supported by the elevated levels of platelet cyclic GMP observed in the presence of PMN [6].

In addition to NO-mediated platelet inhibition, PMN may also control platelet reactivity via NO-independent mechanisms. Zatta et al. [10] reported that a chemically stable compound – besides the previously well characterized labile NO – contributes to PMN-dependent platelet inhibition. In that study the inhibitory effect of PMN on platelet aggregation was also found using whole citrated blood. In agreement with these data, Schattner et al. [11] also observed PMN-mediated platelet inhibition through factor(s) other than arachidonic acid metabolite(s), oxygen radicals, proteases or NO. Furthermore, in an *in vitro* experimental system allowing to evaluate platelet activation and recruitment, releasates from combined suspensions of PMN and platelets demonstrated inhibition of platelet serotonin release and inhibition of platelet recruitment when thrombin or collagen were the agonists. The effects were not attributable to NO-like activity [12]. Platelet ADP removal by ADPase activities expressed by PMN should also be considered [10, 12]. Finally, elastase, a PMN-derived protease, has been shown to prevent thrombin-induced platelet activation through the cleavage of GP Ib [13].

Altogether these data indicate that PMN may inhibit platelet activation by both NO-dependent and NO-independent mechanisms. In conclusion, independent on the mechanisms involved, PMN, under well defined methodologic conditions, can limit platelet activation *in vitro*.

Platelet activation induced by PMN

It has been reported that several PMN-derived products, such as myeloperoxidase, hydrogen peroxide (H_2O_2) and superoxide anion (O_2^-), induce platelet activation [14, 15] and that leukotrienes (C_4, D_4 and E_4) potentiate epinephrine-induced aggregation [16]. However, as these observations have not been repeated in other laboratories, their relevance is questionable.

Platelet Activating Factor (PAF), a lipid mediator produced by PMN, is endowed with platelet stimulating activity [17]. Whether PAF is actually released outside PMN is a matter of controversy [18, 19]. This mediator, which seems to play a role in rabbit PMN-platelet cooperation [20, 21], has not been clearly implicated in PMN-dependent platelet activation with human cells [22].

The involvement of serine proteinases in PMN-dependent platelet activation was first suggested in rabbits, by the observation that diisopropyl fluorophosphate, an inhibitor of proteinases, prevented PMN-dependent platelet activation [23]. A more direct role for proteinases was indicated by the observation that preincubation of platelets with chymotrypsin-like cationic proteins from human granulocytes resulted in enhanced platelet serotonin release initiated by thrombin or by immune complexes [24]. The work by Bykowska *et al.* [25] provided the first direct evidence that a neutral serine proteinase – chymotrypsin-like – purified from human neutrophils was able to stimulate platelet function. This pivotal observation by the Polish group was extended few years later by Chignard *et al.* [26]: these Authors described a potent neutrophil-derived platelet agonist, provisionally called "neutrophilin", which was able to induce platelet activation by involving platelet cytoplasmic Ca^{2+} increase. In subsequent studies "neutrophilin" was identified as cathepsin G [27] and a specific receptor on platelet surface was described [28].

Platelet activation by PMN-derived cathepsin G

Cathepsin G provides a secondary activating signal to platelets after primary PMN activation with formyl-Methionyl-Leucyl-Phenylalanine (fMLP) [26, 29], the activated fifth component of complement (c5a) [30] and most likely with leukotriene B_4 and PAF [31].

Moreover priming of PMN with tumor necrosis factor (TNF), which enhanced cathepsin G release from fMLP-activated PMN, potentiated PMN-dependent platelet activation [32].

In all experiments with human PMN [26, 27, 29–32] cathepsin G was the essential mediator of PMN-induced platelet aggregation, serotonin release and TxA_2 production.

Elastase, through the enzymatic cleavage of GPIIIa on platelet surface, may induce the exposures of active fibrinogen receptors allowing platelet aggregation in the presence of fibrinogen [33]. This is not in contrast with the previously mentioned inhibition of platelet function by elastase [13], because in those experiments platelets were incubated with elastase in the absence of fibrinogen.

All data on PMN-dependent platelet activation were obtained in the presence of cytochalasin B [26, 27, 29–32], which is necessary to allow the release of the content of azurophilic granules from PMN activated by chemotactic factors in suspension [34]. However, the release of the content of azurophilic granules from PMN *in vitro* cannot be considered an artifact due to cytochalasin B, as it has been demonstrated after PMN adhesion to plastic surfaces [35] or during PMN adherence and migration on fibrinogen-coated surfaces [36, 37] or on subendothelial matrix [38]. It has also been demonstrated that PMN, in the absence of cytochalasin B, can release the azurophilic granule content when stimulated by fMLP after 5 min priming with PAF [39].

Biochemistry of cathepsin G-induced platelet activation

The serine proteinase cathepsin G, released by activated polymorphonuclear leukocytes, induces platelet aggregation, serotonin secretion, thromboxane B_2 production and increase of intraplatelet Ca^{2+} levels ($[Ca^{2+}]_i$) all in a concentration dependent manner (50–200 nM). Preventing Ca^{2+} influx with Ni^{2+}, a divalent cation channel inhibitor, cathepsin G-induced $[Ca^{2+}]_i$ rise was inhibited by more than 90%. Quenching of the fluorescence signal obtained by adding Mn^{2+} 3 sec or 3 min after cathepsin G, provided evidence for a rapid and sustained divalent cation channel opening in the platelet membrane. No accumulation of inositol triphosphates could be detected under platelet stimulation by cathepsin G [40]. Inhibition of protein kinase C (PKC) by staurosporine resulted in a decrease of cathepsin G-induced platelet aggregation and serotonin secretion. Cathepsin G also induced a rapid (5 sec) and sustained (5 min) phosphorylation of the PKC substrate (47 kDa protein), indicating that PKC is activated in platelets stimulated by cathepsin G. Moreover this agonist enhanced the binding of [^{3}H] phorbol 12, 13-dibutyrate to intact human platelets, indicating that cathepsin G induces the traslocation of PKC from the cytosol to the platelet plasma membrane. Preincubation of human platelets with staurosporine enhanced, while PMA reduced both Ca^{2+} rises and quenching by Mn^{2+} of fluorescence signal. These results indicate that in platelets: (i) cathepsin G induces $[Ca^{2+}]_i$ increase mainly through an influx across the plasma membrane; (ii) PKC is involved in the signal trasduction induced by cathepsin G; (iii) Ca^{2+} channels opening during activation by cathepsin G may occur under the control of PKC (unpublished observations).

Transcellular metabolism of arachidonic acid in PMN-induced platelet activation

TxB_2 production in platelet/PMN suspensions challenged with 1μM fMLP could not be completely explained by cathepsin G-stimulated platelet arachidonate (AA) metabolism. Indeed the amount of TxB_2 found in supernatants of this experimental system was several times higher than that measured when platelets were stimulated by supernatants from fMLP-activated PMN. This difference did not result from a greater availability of cathepsin G, since PMN release is the same in the presence or absence of platelets [29].

Using ^{3}H-AA-labelled PMN, it was shown that PMN-induced TxB_2 production is the result of transcellular metabolism of AA between fMLP-activated PMN and cathepsin G-stimulated platelets. Analysis of radioactive metabolites of AA demonstrated that metabolization of AA from activated PMN is greater in the presence of platelets and TxB_2 and 12-HHT are synthesized when PMN are activated mixed to unlabelled platelets. TxB_2 formation was completely blocked by aspirin treatment of platelets or by the antiproteinase eglin C preventing cathepsin G-induced platelet activation. All these experiments demonstrate that part of the TxB_2 formed in mixed cell suspensions is the result of a transcellular metabolism in which platelets utilize PMN-derived unmetabolized AA to synthesize TxB_2. The PMN-platelet contact and cathepsin G activation of platelets are the essential conditions for this phenomenon [41].

Pharmacological inhibition of cathepsin G-induced platelet activation

Heparin is a widely used antithrombotic drug both for the prevention and the treatment of venous and arterial thrombosis. The rationale for the use of heparin is based upon its ability to inhibit blood coagulation by enhancing the inhibition of thrombin by antithrombin III. However, whether anticoagulation is fully responsible for the antithrombotic activity of heparin is questionable.

Standard heparin was reported to inhibit the proteinase activity of cathepsin G [42, 43]. Recently Ferrer *et al.* [44] reported that standard and low molecular weight heparin prevent the effect of this proteinase on platelets.

Different heparin preparations inhibit platelet activation induced by cathepsin G released from activated PMN in a mixed cell system, or by the purified enzyme [45]. In the same range of concentrations preventing platelet activation induced by purified cathepsin G, heparins inhibit the proteinase activity of the enzyme. However, in contrast to the complete prevention of the effect of cathepsin G on platelet, the maximal inhibition of the proteinase activity never exceeded 60% of inhibition. This discrepancy could be due to the use for catalytic activity measurements of a small substrate such as N-succinyl-ala-ala-pro-phe-p-nitroanilide; the latter, at variance with the receptor bound to platelet membrane, could maintain some residual access to the catalytic site of cathepsin G. Another possibility is that heparin interacts with cathepsin G at site(s) other than the catalytic site, i.e. a platelet binding site. However, since the stimulatory effect of cathepsin G on platelets depends on the proteinase activity of the enzyme [28] inhibition of cathepsin G catalytic activity by heparins accounts for the inhibitory effect of the drug on cathepsin G-induced platelet activation. The inhibitory effect of heparins on cathepsin G is probably subsequent to the formation of a complex between negatively charged sulfate groups of heparin and the cationic protein [43]. This interaction probably modifies the catalytic site of the enzyme.

Heparins inhibit cathepsin G-induced platelet activation also in a system of mixed platelet/PMN suspensions. The reduced efficacy in this system can be explained by the presence of other proteinases, such as elastase, released by activated PMN, which binds heparin reducing its availability for cathepsin G, or by the formation of a microenvironment between activated PMN and platelets, allowing greater local concentration of cathepsin G. The inhibitory effect of heparins on cathepsin G-induced platelet activation adds a new possible mechanism to the antithrombotic effect of this drug.

More recently inhibition of platelet activation induced by cathepsin G has also been observed with defibrotide, a polydeoxyribonucleotide endowed with antithrombotic effects in different experimental animal models. The inhibitory effect was due to inhibition of the catalytic activity of the enzyme. In the same experimental conditions defibrotide failed to prevent platelet activation by thrombin [46].

PMN-platelet interaction *in vivo*

Although PMN-induced platelet activation through cathepsin G released from azurophilic granules has been so far only demonstrated *in vitro*, we believe that it may occur *in vivo* in conditions favoring thrombosis, in some of which release of the content of azurophilic granules has been shown. In fact, leukocyte elastase release has been shown in the medium during blood coagulation [47], and in plasma from patients with leukemia and septicemia [48]; $\alpha 1$-antitrypsin-elastase complex increased in plasma from patients with disseminated intravascular coagulation [49]. Lately Nuijens *et al.* [50] have provided further evidence that activation and degranulation of neutrophils occurred in patients with sepsis, a condition in which presumably different agonists cooperate in inducing PMN activation. In this study elastase $\alpha 1$-antitrypsin complexes, an index of azurophilic granules content, were inversely related to platelet number.

Increased elastase activity has also been shown in plasma from patients with myocardial infarction [51] indicating leukocyte activation and azurophilic granule release also in this disease. Although cathepsin G is most likely released together with elastase into the circulation in several pathologic conditions, it does not necessarily induce platelet activation. Indeed, plasma antiproteinases are able to immediately block both elastase and cathepsin G activities [52]. However, it has been recently suggested that membrane to membrane contact *in vitro* between PMN and platelets could create a microenvironment in which cathepsin G, discharged from stimulated PMN on adherent platelets, is protected against different antiproteinases [29].

Cell-cell contact is therefore an important aspect of PMN-platelet interaction because it creates optimal conditions for cell-cell communication via soluble mediators.

Platelets and PMN might interact through specific membrane proteins. Indeed activated platelets expose on their surface a protein contained in the membrane of the alpha-granules, called P-selectin, previously known as 'platelet adhesion dependent granule external membrane protein' (PADGEM) [53] or granule membrane protein (GMP–140) [54], that specifically interacts with a glycoprotein (CD 15) on the surface of PMN and monocytes [55]. Cloning of this protein has been recently reported [56].

A P-selectin independent mechanism of PMN-platelet adhesion has also been recently reported [57].

Adhesion between PMN and platelet membranes suggests that maximal effect of mediators during cell-cell interaction can be achieved in a microenvironment limited by the intermembrane adhesion sites. However the importance of a specific, receptor-mediated adhesion step for platelet-PMN functional interaction remains to be established.

Conclusions

The *in vitro* experiments reviewed here demonstrate that in specific experimental conditions, PMN can either inhibit or activate platelets. At present, this discipline is quite controversial. Several and not yet well characterized factors may be involved. These include EDRF/NO, ADPase activities and 15-hydroxy acids of the eicosanoids pathway such as the lipoxins. These may play a role in mediation of PMN-dependent platelet interactions.

The inhibitory effect of PMN may coexist with a potent stimulatory effect when activated-PMN release the content of their azurophilic granules. Cathepsin G, a neutral serine proteinase, is the major mediator of this effect. While convincing data are already available, suggesting PMN-dependent platelet activation *in vivo* in different animal experimental models [58–61], no data are available, to our knowledge, demonstrating PMN-dependent platelet inhibition *in vivo*.

Despite the reported contrasting results on platelet/PMN interactions *in vitro*, a role of such a cell interaction in the pathogenesis of thrombosis is supported by several epidemiological studies: indeed, a positive correlation was found between the number of circulating leukocytes, especially PMN, and the development of ischemic disease (see for review, [62]). More recently the Caerphilly and Speedwell study also indicated white blood cell count as an independent risk factor for ischemic heart disease [63]. However, a cause-effect relationship between PMN number and vascular events has not yet been shown.

Besides platelet activation, other mechanism(s) might explain the contribution of PMN to the development of vascular disease. One of these is endothelial cell injury, mediated by PMN-derived toxic oxygen radicals and/or proteolytic enzymes [64]. Cathepsin G and elastase, by modifying endothelial cell function, might contribute to the development of a prothrombotic state of the endothelial cell: both enzymes may indeed suppress thrombin-induced prostacyclin production [65] and increase the activity of the fibrinolysis inhibitor PAI–1 [66].

Human PMN contain 0.85 ± 0.10 μg of cathepsin G and 1.11 ± 0.14 μg of elastase per 10^6 cells [67], that is a very effective weaponry for inducing platelet activation and affecting endothelial cell function, at least *in vitro*.

Oxidants produced by activated PMN not only directly contribute to endothelial damage but may also damage the methionine-rich active site of α1-proteinase inhibitor, thus reducing the protective potential against PMN-derived proteinases [68].

In conclusion, when considering the effects of PMN on endothelial cells, in addition to the reported PMN-induced platelet activation via cathepsin G, PMN-derived proteinases should be viewed as potential mediators in the pathogenesis of ischemic disease.

Ackowledgements

This work was supported by the National Research Council, Rome, Italy, (Convenzione C.N.R. – Consorzio Mario Negri Sud).

N.M. was on leave of absence from National Academy of Medicine, Buenos Aires, Argentina.

P.P. is the recipient of a fellowship from the Centro di Formazione e Studi per il Mezzogiorno-Formez (Progetto Speciale "Ricerca Scientifica e Applicata nel Mezzogiorno").

References

1. Bizzozero, J., 'Über einen neuen Formbestandteil des Blutes und dessen Rolle bei der Thrombose und Blutgerinnung', *Virchows Arch. Pathol. Anat. Physiol. Klin. Med.* 1882, 90: 261–332.
2. Bazzoni, G., Dejana, E., and Del Maschio, A., 'Platelet-dependent modulation of neutrophil function', *Pharmacol. Res.* 1992, 26: 269–272.
3. Villa, S., Rotilio, D., Donati, M. B., and De Gaetano, G., 'Human blood leukocytes in vitro generate an inhibitor of platelet aggregation', *Thromb. Res.* 1981, 24: 485–487.
4. Vericel, E. and Lagarde, M., '15-hydroxyperoxyeicosatetraenoic acid inhibits human platelet aggregation', *Lipids* 1980, 15: 472–474.
5. Rimele, T. J., Sturm, R. J., Adams, L. M., Henry, D. E., Heaslip, R. J., Weichman, B. M., and Grimes, D., 'Interaction of neutrophils with vascular smooth muscle: identification of a neutrophil-derived relaxing factor', *J. Pharmacol. Exper. Ther.* 1988, 245: 102–111.
6. Salvemini, D., De Nucci, G., Gryglewski, R., and Vane, J. R., 'Human neutrophils and mononuclear cells inhibit platelet aggregation by releasing a nitric oxide-like factor', *Proc. Natl. Acad. Sci. USA* 1989, 86: 6328–6332.
7. McCall, T. B., Boughton-Smith, N. G., Palmer, R. M. J., Whittle, B. J. R., and Moncada, S., 'Synthesis of nitric oxide from L-arginine by neutrophils. Release and interaction with superoxide anion', *Biochem. J.* 1989, 261: 293–296.
8. Nicolini, F. A., Wilson, A. C., Metha, P., and Metha, J. L., 'Comparative platelet inhibitory effects of human neutrophils and lymphocytes', *J. Lab. Clin. Med.* 1990, 116: 147–152.

9. Faint, R. W., Mackie, I. J., and Machin, S. J., 'Platelet aggregation is inhibited by a nitric oxide-like factor released from human neutrophils in vivo', *Br. J. Haematol.* 1991, 77: 539–545.
10. Zatta, A., Prosdocimi, M., Bertelé, V., Bazzoni, G., and Del Maschio, A., 'Inhibition of platelet function by polymorphonuclear leukocytes', *J. Lab. Clin. Med.* 1990, 116: 651–660.
11. Schattner, M. A., Geffner, J. R., Isturiz, M. A., and Lazzari, M. A., 'Inhibition of human platelet activation by polymorphonuclear leukocytes', *Br. J. Pharmacol.* 1990, 101: 253–256.
12. Valles, J., Santos, M. T., Marcus, A. J., Safier, L. B., Broekman, M. J., Islam, N., Ullman, H. L., and Eiroa, A. M., 'Neutrophils inhibit both platelet activation and recruitment', *Clin. Res.* 1990, 38: 232A.
13. Brower, M. S., Levin, R. I., and Garry, K., 'Human neutrophil elastase modulates platelet function by limited proteolysis of membrane glycoproteins', *J. Clin. Invest.* 1985, 75: 657–666.
14. Clark, R. A. and Klebanoff, S. J., 'Neutrophil-platelet interaction mediated by myeloperoxidase and hydrogen peroxide', *J. Immunol.* 1980, 124: 399–405.
15. Handin, R. I., Karabin, R., and Boxer, G. J., 'Enhancement of platelet function by superoxide anion', *J. Clin. Invest.* 1977, 59: 959–965.
16. Mehta, P., Mehta, J., Lawson, D., Krop, I., and Letts, L. G., 'Leukotrienes potentiate the effects of epinephrine and thrombin on human platelet aggregation', *Thromb. Res.* 1986, 41: 731–738.
17. Chignard, M., Keraly, C. L., Nunez, D., Cöeffier, E., and Benveniste, J., 'PAF-acether and platelets', in: *Platelets in Biology and Pathology III*, MacIntyre, D. E., Gordon, J. L. (eds.), Elsevier Science Publishers, Cambridge, 1987, 289–315.
18. Ludwig, J. C., Hoppens, C. L., McManus, L. M., Mott, G. E., and Pinckard, R. N., 'Modulation of platelet activating factor (PAF) synthesis and release from human polymorphonuclear leukocytes (PMN): role of extracellular albumin', *Arch. Biochem. Biophys.* 1985, 241: 337–347.
19. Lynch, J. M. and Henson, P. M., 'The intracellular retention of newly synthesized platelet activating factor', *J. Immunol.* 1986, 137: 2653–2661.
20. Oda, M., Satouchi, K., Yasunaga, K., and Saito, K., 'Polymorphonuclear leukocyte-platelet interactions: acetylglyceryl ether phosphocholine-induced platelet activation under stimulation with chemotactic peptide', *J. Biochem.* 1986, 100: 1117–1123.
21. Cöeffier, E., Joseph, D., Prévost, M.-C., and Vargaftig, B. B., 'Platelet-leukocyte interaction: activation of rabbit platelets by FMLP-stimulated neutrophils', *Br. J. Pharmac.* 1987, 92: 393–406.
22. Virella, G., Espinoza, A., Patrick, H., and Colwell, J. A., 'Polymorphonuclear leucocytes release a factor(s) that induces platelet aggregation and ATP release after interaction with insoluble and surface-fixed immune complexes', *Clin. Exp. Immunol.* 1982, 49: 684–694.
23. Henson, P. M., 'Mechanisms of release of constituents from rabbit platelets by antigen-antibody complexes and complement. II. Interaction of platelets with neutrophils', *J. Immunol.* 1970, 105: 490–501.
24. Hällgren, R. and Venge, P., 'Cationic proteins of human granulocytes. Effects on human platelet aggregation and serotonin release', *Inflammation* 1976, 1: 359–370.
25. Bykowska, K., Kaczanowska, J., Karpowicz, M., Stachurska, J., and Kopec, M., 'Effect of neutral proteases from blood leukocytes on human platelets', *Thromb. Haemost.* 1983', 50: 768–772.
26. Chignard, M., Selak, M. A., and Smith, J. B., 'Direct evidence for the existence of a neutrophilin-derived platelet activator (neutrophilin)', *Proc. Natl. Acad. Sci. USA* 1986, 83: 8609–8613.
27. Selak, M. A., Chignard, M., and Smith, J. B., 'Cathepsin G is a strong platelet agonist released by neutrophils', *Biochem. J.* 1988, 251: 293–299.

28. Selak, M. A. and Smith, J. B., 'Cathepsin G binding to human platelets. Evidence for a specific receptor', *Biochem. J.* 1990, 266: 55–62.
29. Evangelista, V., Rajtar, G., De Gaetano, G., White, J. G., and Cerletti, C., 'Platelet activation by fMLP-stimulated polymorphonuclear leukocytes: the activity of cathepsin G is not prevented by antiproteinases', *Blood* 1991, 77: 2379–2388.
30. Ferrer-Lopez, P., Renesto, P., Schattner, M., Bassot, S., Laurent, P., and Chignard, M., 'Activation of human platelets by C5a-stimulated neutrophils: a role for cathepsin G', *Am. J. Physiol.* 1990, 258: C1100–1107.
31. Del Maschio, A., Evangelista, V., Chen, Z. M., Cerletti, C., and De Gaetano, G., 'Platelet activation induced by polymorphonuclear leukocytes exposed to chemotactic agents', *Am. J. Physiol.* 1990, 258: H870–879.
32. Renesto, P. and Chignard, M., 'Tumor necrosis factor-a enhances platelet activation via cathepsin G released from neutrophils', *J. Immunol.* 1991, 146: 2305–2309.
33. Kornecki, E., Ehrlich, Y. H., Egbring, R., Gramse, M., Seitz, R., Eckardt, A., Lukasiewicz, H., and Niewiarowski, S., 'Granulocyte-platelet interaction and platelet fibrinogen receptor exposure', *Am. J. Physiol.* 1988, 255: H651–658.
34. Bentwood, B. J. and Henson, P. M., 'The sequential release of granule constituents from human neutrophils', *J. Immunol.* 1980, 124: 855–862.
35. Schleiffenbaum, B., Moser, R., Patarroyo, M., and Fehr, J., 'The cell surface glycoprotein Mac–1 (CD1b/CD18) mediates neutrophil adhesion and modulates degranulation independently of its quantitative cell surface expression', *J. Immunol.* 1989, 142: 3537–3545.
36. Weitz, J. I., Huang, A. J., Landman, S. L., Nicholson, S. C., and Silverstein, S. C., 'Elastase-mediated fibrinogenolysis by chemoattractant-stimulated neutrophils occurs in the presence of physiologic concentrations of antiproteinases', *J. Exp. Med.* 1987, 166: 1836–1850.
37. Wright, S. D., Weitz, J. I., Huang, A. J., Levin, S. M., and Silverstein, S. C., 'Complement receptor type three (CD11b/CD18) of human polymorphonuclear leukocytes recognizes fibrinogen', *Proc. Natl. Acad. Sci. USA* 1988, 85: 7734–7738.
38. Weiss, S. J. and Regiani, S., 'Neutrophils degrade subendothelial matrices in the presence of alpha–1-proteinase inhibitor. Cooperative use of lysosomal proteinases and oxygen metabolites', *J. Clin. Invest.* 1984, 73: 1297–1303.
39. Vercellotti, G. M., Yin, H. Q., Gustafson, K. S., Nelson, R. D., and Jacob, H. S., 'Platelet-activating factor primes neutrophil responses to agonists: role in promoting neutrophil-mediated endothelial damage', *Blood* 1988, 71: 1100–1107.
40. Molino, M., Di Lallo, M., De Gaetano, G., and Cerletti, C., 'Intracellular Ca^{2+} rise in human platelets by polymorphonuclear leucocyte-derived cathepsin G', *Biochem. J.* 1992, 288: 741–745.
41. Maugeri, N., Evangelista, V., Piccardoni, P., Dell'Elba, G., Celardo, A., De Gaetano, G., and Cerletti, C., 'Transcellular metabolism of arachidonic acid: increased platelet thromboxane generation in the presence of activated polymorphonuclear leukocytes', *Blood* 1992, 80: 447–451.
42. Marossy, M., 'Interaction of the chymotrypsin- and elastase-like enzymes of the human granulocyte with glycosaminoglycans', *Biochim. Biophys. Acta* 1981, 659: 351–361.
43. Redini, F., Tixier, J. M., Petitou, M., Choay, J., Roberts, L., and Hornebeck, W., 'Inhibition of leukocytes elastase by heparin and its derivatives', *Biochem. J.* 1988, 252: 515–519.
44. Ferrer, P., Renesto, P., and Chignard, M., 'Inhibition by heparin of platelet activation by human neutrophil-derived cathepsin G', *Am. Rev. Resp. Dis.* 1990, 141: A109.
45. Evangelista, V., Piccardoni, P., Maugeri, N., De Gaetano, G., and Cerletti, C., 'Inhibition by heparin of platelet activation induced by neutrophil-derived cathepsin G', *Eur. J. Pharmacol.* 1992, 216: 401–405.
46. Evangelista, V., Piccardoni, P., De Gaetano, G., and Cerletti, C., 'Defibrotide inhibits platelet activation by cathepsin G released from stimulated polymorphonuclear leukocytes', *Thromb. Haemostas.* 1992, 67: 660–664.
47. Plow, E. F., 'Leukocyte elastase release during blood coagulation. A potential mechanism

for activation of the alternative fibrinolytic pathway', *J. Clin. Invest.* 1982, 69: 564–572.
48. Egbring, R., Schmidt, W., Fuchs, G., and Havemann, K., 'Demonstration of granulocytic proteases in plasma of patients with acute leukemia and septicemia with coagulation defects', *Blood* 1977, 49: 219–231.
49. Brower, M. S. and Harpel, P. C., 'Alpha–1-antitrypsin-human leukocyte elastase complexes in blood: quantification by an enzyme-linked differential antibody immunosorbent assay and comparison with alpha–2-plasmin inhibitor-plasmin complex', *Blood* 1983, 61: 842–849.
50. Nuijens, J. H., Abbink, J. J., Wachtfogel, Y. T., Colman, R. W., Eerenberg, A. J. M., Dors, D., Kamp, A. J. M., Strack van Schijndel, R. J. M., Thijs, L. G., and Hack, C. E., 'Plasma elastase α1-antitrypsin and lactoferrin in sepsis: evidence for neutrophils as mediators in fatal sepsis', *J. Lab. Clin. Med.* 1992, 119: 159:68.
51. Mehta, J., Dinerman, J., Mehta, P., Saldeen, T. G. P., Lawson, D., Donnelly, W. H., and Wallin, R., 'Neutrophil function in ischemic heart disease', *Circulation* 1989, 79: 549–556.
52. Travis, J. and Salveson, G. S., 'Human plasma proteinase inhibitors', *Ann. Rev. Biochem.* 1983, 52: 655–709.
53. Larsen, E., Celi, A., Gilbert, G. E., Furie, B. C., Erban, J. K., Bonfanti, R., Wagner, D. D., and Furie, B., 'PADGEM protein: a receptor that mediates the interaction of activated platelets with neutrophils and monocytes', *Cell* 1989, 59: 305–312.
54. Hamburger, S. A. and McEver, R. P., 'GMP–140 mediates adhesion of stimulated platelets to neutrophils', *Blood* 1990, 75: 550–554.
55. Larsen, E., Palabrica, T., Sajer, S., Gilbert, G. E., Wagner, D. D., Furie, B. C., and Furie, B., 'PADGEM-dependent adhesion of platelets to monocytes and neutrophils is mediated by a lineage-specific carbohydrate, LNF III (CD15)', *Cell* 1990, 63: 467–474.
56. Johnston, G. I., Cook, R. G., and McEver, R. P., 'Cloning of GMP–140, a granule membrane protein of platelets and endothelium: sequence similarity to proteins involved in cell adhesion and inflammation', *Cell* 1989, 56: 1033–1044.
57. Rinder, H. M., Bonan, J. L., Rinder, C. S., Ault, K. A., and Smith, B. R., 'Activated and unactivated platelet adhesion to monocytes and neutrophils', *Blood* 1991, 78: 1760–1769.
58. Issekutz, A. C., Ripley, M., and Jackson, J. R., 'Role of neutrophils in the deposition of platelets during acute inflammation', *Lab. Invest.* 1983, 49: 716–724.
59. Schaub, R. G., Simmons, C. A., Koets, M. H., Romano, P. J. II, and Stewart, G. J., 'Early events in the formation of a venous thrombus following local trauma and stasis', *Lab. Invest.* 1984, 51: 218–224.
60. Bednar, M., Smith, B., Pinto, A., and Mullane, K. M., 'Neutrophil depletion suppresses ^{111}In-labeled platelet accumulation in infarcted myocardium', *J. Cardiovasc. Pharmacol.* 1985, 7: 906–912.
61. Johnson, R. J., Alpers, C. E., Pritzl, P., Schulze, M., Baker, P., Pruchno, C., and Couser, W. G., 'Platelets mediate neutrophil-dependent immune complex nephritis in the rat', *J. Clin. Invest.* 1988, 82: 1225–1235.
62. Ernst, E., Hammerschmidt, D. E., Bagge, U., Matrai, A., and Dormandy, J. A., 'Leukocytes and the risk of ischemic diseases', *JAMA* 1987, 257: 2318–2324.
63. Yarnell, J. W. G., Baker, I. A., Sweetnam, P. M., Bainton, D., O'Brien, J. R., Whitehead, P. J., and Elwood, P. C., 'Fibrinogen, viscosity, and white blood cell count are major risk factors for ischemic hearth disease. The Caerphilly and Speedwell Collaborative Hearth Disease Studies', *Circulation* 1991, 83: 836–844.
64. Harlan, J. M., 'Leukocyte-endothelial interactions', *Blood* 1985, 65: 513–525.
65. Weksler, B. B., Jaffe, E. A., Brower, M. S., and Cole, O. F., 'Human leukocyte cathepsin G and elastase specifically suppress thrombin-induced prostacyclin production in human endothelial cells', *Blood* 1989, 74: 1627–1634.
66. Pintucci, P., Iacoviello, L., Amore, C., Evangelista, V., Cerletti, C., and Donati, M. B., 'Cathepsin G-induced release of PAI–1 from platelets and endothelial cells: a new thrombogenic property of PMN?', *Blood* 1991, 78: 397a.

67. Campbell, E. J., Silverman, E. K., and Campbell, M. A., 'Elastase and cathepsin G of human monocytes. Quantification of cellular content, release in response to stimuli, and heterogeneity in elastase-mediated proteolytic activity', *J. Immunol.* 1989, 143: 2961–2968.
68. Weiss, S. J., 'Tissue destruction by neutrophils', *N. Engl. J. Med.* 1989, 320: 365–376.

PART THREE

Discussion chapters

9. Platelet collection, storage and transfusion

Davies: We have three suggestions for this evening's discussion and I think it would be useful to start with the first item that is on the programme, "How to keep platelet function intact during storage before platelet transfusion". One of the slides that you showed, Jean-Luc was useful in starting the discussion. You posed some of the questions that relate to platelet preservation and storage. But one of the first things that we could talk about, is to start right at the beginning and discuss whether we should express a preference for one or other method of platelet collection. The present methods are either by plasmapheresis in which there is a much better yield and you return the blood products to the donor, or by wide-bore needle venepuncture and collection of blood into a bag. Clearly any way that you get blood out of the circulation is going to cause activation of coagulation and platelet activation.

Jean-Luc do you have any practical experience of plasmapheresis?

Wautier: Yes, well I think when you are a haematologist you prefer to transfuse a patient with platelet which is collected by plasmapheresis. Firstly, because you have platelets only from one donor so you minimise the risk of all-immunisation. Secondly, most of the time we use platelets which have been collected in the previous 24 hr and not stored for 3–4 days, and the third thing is that using platelets coming onl y from donor you also minimise the risk of contamination by viruses. Obviously there are some tests which are available but we know that there are still some viruses that we are not able to detect or some which we are unable to detect at the present time so we know that instead of having ten donors, having one donor would reduce the risk. I think all these reasons are in favour of having platelets coming from one donor collected by plasmapheresis. The arguments against this type of collection are that it is more expensive, because we have to use a very expensive machine to collect the platelets, the second that all the systems, the collecting systems, the tubing and the bags are more expensive than the bags which are used for standard collections, arguments which are against plasmapheresis.

Davies: Does anyone else have any experience with plasmapheresis or any thoughts about it or other methods of collection?

Hanson: I have a minor negative comment. Some of the more commonly

Y. F. Missirlis and J.-L. Wautier (eds.), The Role of Platelets in Blood-Biomaterial Interactions, 109–121.

used plasmapheresis devices in the United States are not without problems of accumulation of platelets and blood elements, particularly in the inflow lines. Also, since platelets are collected in acid citrate dextrose, there has been the occasional problem of excessive citrate burden in individual patients with adverse reactions. While I do not think these minor concerns outweigh the many positive aspects, plasmapheresis is not without some occasional problems.

Ordinas: I think that with regard to the strategy of blood centers, it depends on each Hospital. For example, in our hospital the blood bank is relatively small for the big hospital that it is, with 1,000 beds including a program for bone marrow and liver transplantation which require both systems: the pool platelets and typed single donor platelets. In cases with leukemia, alloimmuniztion is not always so important since, when these patients bleed, the principal objective is to arrest the bleeding and therefore, in these patients, pool platelets are useful. In special situations,however, it would be more useful to have a program of typed single donor platelets.

Currently our group is interested in the role of platelet transfusion in the stopping of bleeding episodes in hematologic patients. We are aware that in most patients the stopping of the bleeding episode is related to the generation of thrombin *in vivo*, formation of fibrin, and consequently, the formation of the hemostatic plug. We have published that, using the Baumgartner perfusion system , when you perfuse blood from patients with a platelet count of around 15,000, no platelet deposition may be observed on the subendothelium. However, when you begin to transfuse these patients with pool platelets even if they are not compatible, the perfusion is then repeated and even if the platelet count does not increase, the formation of fibrin may be seen on the subendothelium. Thus, meaning the same thing probably happens *in vivo* and what is required to stop bleeding is the generation of thrmobin and formation of fibrin.

In the near future, the strategy for providing platelets for the treatment of such patients by some blood banks involve another type of material for transfusion in these patients.

Davies: What is the active haemostatic constituent do you think? Are you just providing a lipid biolayer and would a lipid micelle perhaps substitute for that?

Ordinas: Yes.

Wautier: I would just say that a freezed dry product prepared with platelets was infused in patients. It has been marketed more than 20 years ago in Germany as a haemostatic product, and I don't know if it is still on the market but there was a meeting in, I guess 1974–75 organised by M. Verstraete in Belgium with a large panel of experts evaluate haemostatic products which were present all through the world at that time and far as I remember this one was not the most efficient in stopping bleeding. There is no real demonstration of the clinical efficacy of this drug as this is the case for many products which were marketed at that time to be haemostatic. So I think we have to be careful when we say that such products has really some efficiency in stopping bleeding in the absence of controlled trials. We can compare this product versus some other products in patients who are thrombocytopaenic. I think there is a real need to have well conducted trials to evaluate the risk and the benefit of the different ways of preparing platelets which are transfused.

Missirlis: Has the biological activity of platelets that have been preserved for one or two or three or four days been evaluated, and how has it been evaluated?

Mulvihill: Yes we have in our laboratory performed evaluation of different bags for platelet storage, different types of biomaterial bags. We carried out a number of tests day by day over a period of up to 5 days on the platelets. Generally, results were a function of the pH which we found to be a very good guide, correlating well with most of the other parameters we tested as to the quality of the platelets. Aggregation tests, in particular to ADP, collagen and thrombin: we found that sometimes there would be almost a peak as if the platelets were activated after a period of one or two days storage and reacted more strongly to ADP, thrombin and collagen. This was followed by a very rapid fall off at day 3 or 4. Thus the platelets changed over the storage time, became activated and perhaps released granule contents and then became less effective from that time onwards. We did not carry out re-injection and radiolabelled control of platelet disappearance from the circulation system, which has been done by other groups. However, platelet activation was one of the interesting points we found. One might consider that slightly activated platelets in the situation where you wish to stop bleeding may not be such a bad thing and that they are going to do their job in blocking the site of injury by reacting quickly to form the haemostatic plug where it is needed. If they do not survive very long in the circulation this is not such a problem. So perhaps platelet quality in storage is less important. One other thing I might say with regard to plasmapheresis circuits and platelets, we noticed like Mr Hanson that sometimes the blood filters on the inlet lines would contain platelet-fibrin thrombi, particularly when we were dealing with plasmapheresis in patients with immunoglobulin disorders. Perhaps immunoglobulin deposed on the blood lines and artificial surfaces tended to cause thrombus formation. We were reduced at one stage to albumin passivation of these surfaces, including the entire blood line, to reduce the reactivity towards platelets, otherwise we would sometimes find the system completely blocked with platelet-fibrin thrombi. Hence there is certainly a considerable degree of platelet activation in this kind of system.

Davies: Before we discuss bags and preservatives and so on, I guess the reality is that most organisations are going to settle, as Dr. Ordinas has said, for a combination of plasmapheresis and classical methods of platelet collection, just because of the logistics and possibly the expense. But I wanted to ask people with experience whether it is more difficult to get volunteers to donate for plasmapheresis than it is for routine collection. I do not know whether there is a donor problem?

Ordinas: In our experience, we have had no difficulty in organizing a panel of single donors for platelet pheresis since our program was initiated with relatives of patients undergoing bone marrow transplantation. At present, we have 250 donors, who are perfectly HLA typed.

Davies: And they enjoy this role do they?

Ordinas: Yes, they do; so much, in fact, that some have been included in an international registry for bone marrow donors.

Davies: Why do we use citrate in plasmapheresis machines?

Wautier: Not many anticoagulants have been used. Everybody knowing that heparin is terrible. It activates platelets and cannot be used at all and in the system. There could be some accumulation of platelets in the filter. The accumulation of platelets is more often seen in patients that are treated by plasma exchange. What Mrs Mulvihill told us is true. It's less frequent in normal donors but it's also true that sometimes a certain amount of citrate is a problem. The citrate which is used has been based on in-vitro study of the F. Mustard Group that is composed of citric, acid, citrate, dextrose was one which was the best to keep platelets in a nonactive state. So that's the reason this one has been mostly used. Very little has been studied on the use of other additive to collect platelets in this system.

Davies: Any experience with adding PGI_2?

Wautier: The problem is that in the organisation of transfusion itself, the regulation is very strict, you cannot infuse products which are not being approved by all regulation of the country and the only product which has been approved up to now is derivative from ACD. No other additive.

Davies: Anyone have any last thoughts on collection before we go onto bags and preservation in the bags once the platelets are being stored? Perhaps we could go into that. Juliette, you referred earlier to work that you'd done on different kinds of bag composition. Can you expand on what you were saying?

Mulvihill: Yes, we were largely interested in PVC bags with different plastifiers added to them. In particular DEHP which has been traditionally used and a trimellitate plastifier. We did find the trimellitate bags seemed to be better on the whole, particularly after about 3 days. In the standard PVC bags there would be a marked drop in platelet activity whereas the others would tend to hold out to day 4 or 5. We did not test any of the polyolefine bags which have also been on the market for some while, as we mainly tested plastifiers for the basic PVC material. This was because the particular company we were working with at the time marketed these bags and they were interested in the effects of plastifiers on the bags.

Missirlis: Juliette, when you made those tests, did you have the exact specifications of the material, that the bag was made of from the different batches? For example, the amount and type of the contained plasticizer? Or, maybe, each batch was slightly different from an other?

Mulvihill: No, at the time we did these studies the bags were just a code number so it was a blind test, but afterwards we were told the exact percentage of plastifier and the ingredients of the polymer mixture. Thus we did later know the exact composition of the polymers used.

Missirlis: And do you think that measured differences might be due to leakage of plasticizers into the medium?

Mulvihill: As regards platelet quality, I would have my doubts if this would greatly affect it. Leakage of the plastifier does not generally have immediate systemic effects and even in the long term perspective damage to the patient rather than to the quality of the stored platelets has always been the complaint raised against plastifiers. They can be damaging, particularly with repeated infusion of stored platelets. We did find nevertheless that the trimellitate bags were better for preserving platelets, but this could be a question of better gas exchange.

Wautier: Yes but we did not for the same experience as you. We have conducted a study to compare the different functions of platelets stored with or without antiproteases and we had bags and we were never able to get the exact composition of the bags from the manufacturers. They tell us it's a "secret of fabrication" or we cannot tell you that is the exact composition.

Missirlis: Jean-Luc have you done any surface analysis of your bags to see what is on the surface of the bags?

Wautier: No the purpose of our study was to compare if we had better condition of storage with or without antiproteases so that was not the purpose of our study. But we asked the manufacturer and they say we cannot answer your question, its a secret.

Davies: I would guess that it is an area of fairly restricted interest but I must say that in casual reading in the field of transfusion, because it's not a field that I work in, I have seen few papers about the type of bag and what should be the factors that determine what the bag is made of. And I guess that it's mainly simple economics and that people go for the cheapest bags. Does anyone have practical information, other than Juliette, about studies on the type of bag?

Hanson: I recall an early study in which several types of PVC bags from several manufacturers were compared with respect to the lifespan of radiolabelled platelets following transfusion back into patients. Apparently, in those early studies bags of different manufacture did affect platelet survival and it was ultimately resolved to use a certain type of PVC which gave the best result in terms of preserving the platelet lifespan. I am uncertain as to whether or not the properties of the bags currently used are still a limiting factor, or whether reduced platelet lifespan and poor platelet quality is more related to limited gas exchange and the agents added to preserve platelet metabolism. So, I'm not aware of current data showing that the quality of the bags is still an important issue, or of studies in which the blood contacting surfaces have been carefully characterized and related to platelet viability.

Davies: That begs the question how you would actually measure the effect of the bags. We're talking tomorrow in one of the sessions about measuring platelet function, and I don't suppose it is sensible to get into that now but if anyone were going to set up studies looking at the bags or different methods of collection and so on, one of the things you have to decide is what platelet functions should be measured. Clearly doing platelet survival, whatever you think about what platelet survival is actually telling you, is a very complex method of assessing platelet function and if you were doing any sort of extensive study, one would have to look for simpler measurements along the lines that Juliette has indicated.

Mulvihill: These tests we did in the laboratory are certainly simpler, but on the other hand survival tests are more closely related to the clinical situation. Re-injection is probably closer to the actual situation of platelets which are injected or transfused to someone and it is sometimes difficult to correlate the *in vitro* tests with survival tests and clinical trials, not that I know of any work where people, just as Mr Hansen said, have actually tried to compare bag quality in clinical trials. I think in the early days there were quite a number of groups who used *in vitro* tests and possibly platelet survival studies to evaluate the polyolefine bags when they first came onto the market as compared to the traditional PVC bags. It was thought to be a question largely of gas exchange and lower accumulation of lactate in polyolefine bags. Stronger survival in the so-called 5–7 day bags which came onto the market was compared to weaker survival in the 3–5 day bags which had been used up until then. After these early tests interest shifted to the medium, collection techniques and other factors which indeed could be more important in the long run. Most of these studies of bag type were fairly early on in the history of platelet storage.

Hanson: I would add one comment about platelet survival. In our hands this has been a very sensitive measure of platelet function. Following transfusion, platelet survival measurements also provide information about the economy of the transfused cells, in other words, how many platelets circulate and for what period of time. This is probably important when considering multiple transfusions in severely thrombocytopaenic individuals.

Davies: Yes, I accept that platelet survival is telling you something. You say that it relates to other indices of platelet function and so I would ask you whether it is not easier, in practical terms, to do some other analyses of platelet function?

The problem of platelet survival is that it is a very cumbersome technique and there is disagreement as to the best ways of doing it and what it is you are measuring. I would ask this group, which has a lot of experience, whether you have any evidence that you can get good survival in non-functioning platelets under certain circumstances.

Hanson: Other tests of platelet function can of course be performed. In thrombocytopaenia, platelet haemostatic competence is shown by the arrest of bleeding, and the survival of transfused platelets can be estimated from serial platelet counts. *In vitro*, additional tests of platelet function can also be performed, and perhaps correlated with *in vivo* outcomes. It is also possible that dysfunctional platelets could exhibit good platelet survival under some circumstances, but I have no information on this point.

Davies: Well I guess we'll come back to that tomorrow evening. There are a whole lot of considerations which Jean-Luc showed this morning in relation to the preservative fluid, and fluid-gas exchange within the bag and so on. Would you like to recap on that briefly?

Wautier: It is probably not very useful just to go over it because that won't be the paper that we have prepared but there is a few things that I want to add to that. So we are with platelets in the situation where there is a great demand for patients who are thrombocytopaenic for various reasons, for chemotheapy, leukemia, aplasia, or cancer or other primitive thrombocytopaenia and so there is still need for platelet transfusion and there are very little studies which define properly what are the best conditions to keeping function of platelets. There is some guarantee, that the pH is not varying too much, that the bacterial contamination is limited by the new system. That the delay to keep the platelets is limited all these things have been well defined but if the haemostatic function of platelets are kept, we don't know exactly, how long they are kept in good condition? The clinical experience is that platelets which are transfused in the 24 hr following the collection are most of the time more efficient in terms of haemostatic function and when we are looking at some *in vitro* parameters some of the parameters are kept longer.

One more point is when you want to compare different conditions of storing platelets you need a huge amount of platelets at the beginning. You have platelets coming from different donors which have not exactly the same properties, so you should have a huge number of experiments to minimize variation between one donor and the other. I think that was one of the limitations why so little attention has been taken to the function of platelet which are used for transfusion, besides economical point but it is minimal. Millions of platelet which are transfused in patient and I think that's not only an economical problem, it is really a problem to know what product we are using and what is the effect. We spoke this morning about leukocyte and it is obvious that the leukocyte contamination in platelets concentrate is very important. Less leukocyte probably the better the platelets are preserved. There are several things like that which are probably true but have to be really demonstrated by studies that are scientifically performed and not just by the impression of there is a lot of very expensive experiments which are done on platelets in thrombotic disorders and very little attention is given to what are the function of platelets that are transfused.

Davies: I'm sure that's right. You referred very briefly to the work that you'd done with protease inhibitors though you didn't tell us what the outcomes were.

Wautier: We were a little disappointed because we expected that there was mostly proteases coming from leukocytes that could modify platelet glycoprotein or platelet function. We did not find a significant difference in terms of preservation. We found a difference in the preservation of glycoprotein 1b in the first days but no longer than that. So that means that probably it could be good to have some protease inhibitors, possibly more than one because they are not as large as we know and that probably could be of interest to be done. The experiment we did showed that there is a little improvement but not as big as we can expect.

Davies: Well, I don't know whether anyone else has any other thoughts on transfusion.

Mulvihill: Just to confirm the observation about GPIb, we also did electrophoresis studies of the membrane proteins of these platelets. We found that GPIIb/IIIa was relatively stable although we never used protease inhibitors, but GPIb after about 1 or a maximum of 2 days was completely degraded, disappearing very quickly. It seemed to be the most labile of the large group of membrane proteins. So perhaps inhibitors could be useful, but you say you did not observe a great improvement with protease inhibitors in the conservation of GPIb.

Wautier: There was improvement in the first two days and after that there is no major difference.

Ordinas: I think that it is always important to keep in mind that what happens *in vitro* is not always so *in vivo*. For example, if you study platelet aggregation on platelets stored for 5 days, these platelets may respond very badly to any agonist, but if transfused to a patient during a bleeding episode, the bleeding may be stopped. At this point, we go back to my first comment that what is of importance is not the platelet function but rather the initiation of coagulation cascade to form fibrin in the wound.

Davies: My views are similar to yours. I would be interested to know the survival time in the circulation of your 5 day old platelets, that don't react to ADP and so on. I would guess that their survival would alos be short, even though they appear to have some effect in the patient. We're back to the point that Jean-Luc made, that anecdotal experience, while it can be comforting, can also be misleading. One needs to evaluate these things in a more formal way.

This comes back to the difficulties we have in all platelet work in knowing whether any of the things we measure have much to do with what platelets actually do when they're in the circulation.

Wautier: But I disagree with Dr. Ordinas and also I will be myself interested in something. If we insert into liposome some of the glycoproteins of platelets do we have some haemostatic effect?

Ordinas: I do not know. What we need to do is to wait until some pharmaceutical company is willing to promote this kind of project or produce a product related to the same.

Wautier: We know that. There is some experiments which have been presented that when you insert into the liposome the GPIIb/IIa complex and you put two of these liposomes together and you have all the proteins which can bridge one or the other you can also bridge or not?

Kieffer: I don't recollect whether these experiments have been performed. However, it is known that GPIIb-IIIa incorporated onto the surface of phosphatidylcholine vesicles interacts with soluble fibrinogen and that this interaction can be inhibited with a monoclonal antibody to GPIIb-IIIa or with a RGD-containing peptide.

Hanson: There are recently reported studies in which RGD (Arg-Gly-Asp) containing peptides were covalently bound to red cells to create so-called thrombo-erythrocytes. These thrombo-erythrocytes form mixed aggregates with platelets, and could perhaps substitute for platelets if they exhibit good cooperative interactions with the reduced numbers of residual autologous platelets as are present in thrombocytopaenia. However, only *in vitro* studies have been reported to date.

Missirlis: Well, I was just left a little bit confused hearing that old platelets do function and at the same time the idea that if you give phospholipid surfaces to the bleeding patient again it works.

Ordinas: No, this is not correct. The phospholipid idea is just a theory and my impression is that it is only a theory extrapolating the results we found *in vitro* but they could occur *in vivo*. What is true however, is that if you give pool platelets, even if the function of these platelets *in vitro* is not excellent, to a patient bleeding you may eventually stop the bleeding.

Cerletti: I have a comment about the testing of platelet to see if they function. Many years ago Scott Martin published a work in which, if I remember correctly, showed that platelets preserved for a number of days did not respond to arachidonic acid, to ADP, but were able to respond to a couple of aggregating agents, I think it was arachidonic acid and adrenaline, or adrenaline and PAS. So maybe we are testing platelet function not in the most correct or useful way before deciding that platelets do not work.

Wautier: In old works Reimers showed in animals he can take the platelets stimulate the platelets with thrombin, the platelets were completely degranulated. These platelets were transfused into normal rabbits and the platelet recovered their granules and they become active as they were before. So I think some platelet functions wich are lost in the storage conditions can possibly be recovered in *in vivo* situations. Also, possibly the body itself selects the good platelets and the bad platelets and all these good platelets circulate. There are a number of them that are but we know also that in thrombocytopaenic patients with the same number of platelets patients bleed and the other has no haemorrhagic event. So I don't know if this could explain all the different situations we can have in clinich, but that may warn them.

Hanson: I'd like to add one more point about platelet storage. In normal humans platelets may have a finite lifespan of approximately 10 days. Most platelets, probably 80–90% in normal individuals, eventually reach an age of about 10 days and are then cleared from the circulation through a process of platelet senescence. In other words, most platelets probably die of old age although we don't fully understand the mechanisms whereby platelets are recognized as senescent. Thus if platelets initially having a normal age distribution in the range of 0–10 days are stored for 5 days they may continue to age and senesce *in vitro*. If those platelets are then transfused, approximately half, those platelets now having ages greater than 10 days, may be cleared quickly while the remaining half of the initial population, those cells now having ages of 5–10 days, will exhibit a lifespan of about 5 days and a half-life of 2–3 days. Thus, due to *in vitro* aging of platelets, the lifespan of 5 day stored platelets may be no more than about 5 days even if all other platelet functions were perfectly maintained. It would be unreasonable, I think, to expect any bag or storage conditions to maintain platelet function and lifespan indefinitely. That would argue that you've interrupted all the normal metabolic processes and membrane changes that lead to platelet senescence. So, the storage time may have an upper limit of about 5 days, and may always be inversely related to platelet survival and recovery even under optimal conditions.

Davies: Well, we seem to have produced more questions than answers as usual which is probably a good point at which to start thinking about platelet consumption during extracorporeal circulation. You have more experience than any of us, Steve.

Hanson: We have collaborated on animal and clinical studies to try and understand the occasional but serious bleeding tendency that develops in some patients on bypass. One approach tried, that of using regional infusions of prostacyclin into the bypass circuit, worked very nicely in primates to prevent the prolongation in bleeding time and drop in platelet count that was seen in control studies. The same study in clinical patients was without success, perhaps because we were unable to give sufficient amounts of prostacyclin without producing hypotension. So, at this point we don't have a good explanation for the platelet defect that develops during bypass.

Davies: Who has thoughts on this? I was going to ask whether with hollow fibre renal dialysis, you saw the same drop in platelet count that you see with flat bed dialysers.

Hanson: Dialysis seems to be substantially more benign than bypass in terms of platelet destruction and severe bleeding.

Davies: But with the flat bed dialysers you always see this small drop in platellet count?

Hanson: The new hollow fibre dialyzers are better, although early hollow fibre dialyzers could also produce a drop in the platelet count. More recently, dialyzers containing fibers composed of polysulfones have been remarkably nonthrombogenic in animal studies with only standard heparin anticoagulation.

Davies: Does anyone know what this initial drop in platelet count is due to? Where do the platelets go? Are they rapidly made senescent or can you account for them through the loss in the dialyser?

Hanson: Much of the loss can be accounted for by platelet deposition onto the dialyzer. We and others have have labelled platelets with gamma-emitting radioisotopes, and then measured platelet deposition by scintillation camera imaging. We clearly see substantial early platelet accumulations that can change over time due to loss of platelet aggregates by embolization and lysis. Clearly, there is in many cases a very active local consumption of platelets by these devices.

Mulvihill: We studied hollow fibre dialysers in *ex vivo* tests as opposed to animal studies. One test we used to check for platelet aggregation was bTG release and this correlated in fact, not with platelet consumption but with coagulation activation and hollow fibre type. Particularly when using polysulphones, there was very little platelet consumption, a slight decline over a half hour period, but activation of the coagulation system in this case correlated very nicely with platelet bTG release, indicating that a lot of the platelet activation was due to thrombin generation. These two factors could likewise correlate together in a system where the blood is recirculated, for example in an animal model. In some of the early dialysers employing cuprophan membranes which are known to activate complement, there was a certain amount of sequestration in the lungs, especially over the first 10–15 min. This is also relevant to the discussion we had this morning about activation of platelets by complement and coagulation factors and *vice versa*. Did you detect any platelet aggregates in the lungs, in connection with this phenomenon?

Hanson: I'm afraid we didn't look for that.

Mulvihill: This could possibly account for the initial drop.

Hanson: It could indeed. In fact, using bypass apparatus if the blood is returned to the venous system we see a striking transient accumulation of platelet aggregates in the lungs by radioisotope imaging. This could happen to some extent with dialyzers as well.

Davies: It's my understanding though I don't work in any of these fields, that with modern dialysis equipment or modern haemoperfusion systems and cardiac bypass equipment, it is rare to have a significant bleeding problem in a patient. I don't know whether any of the bioengineers have any comments.

Missirlis: Well, I was trying to put the question rather than the answer. If you take the bypass and the haemodialysis systems, since the haemodynamics are totally different in the two systems, and the surfaces (area and geometry) are different, how much is the influence of the surface or the shear on the destruction or the sequestration of platelets?

Ordinas: Also the patient is different. This is also very important.

Davies: Yes I think that's a good point, that in renal dialysis you're dealing with people who have impaired haemostasis, so coagulation is less of a problem. But, as I understand it, you can in an emergency dialyse patients with a hollow fibre dialyser without using any anticoagulant at all. So the haemostatic defect that you produce with a modern hollow fibre dialyser is very small in patients with renal failure. Whereas clearly the stress of the extracorporeal circuit with coronary bypass is very much greater and,as I understand it, that's largely due to the oxygenator.

Hanson: Well, it's certainly a complicated issue. Bypass is generally viewed as the most serious challenge to the haemostatic system because you have exposure of very large surface areas and a complex circuit containing an oxygenator, pump, blood warmer, and various catheters and tubings. Due to these multiple surfaces and devices, which introduce complicated haemodynamic regimes, a fraction of patients develop bleeding problems and other complications which include not only depletion of platelets and fibrinogen but activation of complement, activation and depletion of leukocytes, and so forth. These factors also limit the duration of bypass procedures.

Missirlis: Did I understand well that you can perform dialysis for some hours without anticoagulants?

Davies: Well my remark is hearsay, it doesn't come from practical experience, but I understand from our renal physicians that you can do emergency, short-term dialysis in patients who've got a serious bleeding disorder without using anticoagulation. But of course we're talking of patients, as has been mentioned already, who have a haemostatic defect. So you are not comparing like with like if you're trying to make some comparison with putting people on cardiac bypass.

10. Platelet: haemostasis and anticoagulation

Mulvihill: One of the big problems is the haematocrit which is generally low, lower than 10%. Due to haemodynamic factors this reduces platelet adhesion. After 6 months of erythropoietin treatment to increase the haematocrit in these patients, the authors performed perfusion chamber experiments with the uraemic blood and found that adhesion was almost restored to normal, whilst haematocrit was back to normal. Of course once they ceased the treatment the platelet adhesion dropped off again, so it possibly could be the result of changes in platelet membrane structure and that the platelets themselves were abnormal, but possibly also a haemodynamic effect due to the lower red blood cell count.

Davies: There was a clinical observation from some years ago that if you transfused patients in renal failure with packed red blood cells which didn't have platelets in them you actually improved haemostatic function quite considerably.

Wautier: In the system which has been used by Jean-Pierre Cazenave also the presence of blood cells are needed ; in the absence of red cells you don't have the adhesion up to certain haematocrit there is a relationship between the haematocrit and the platelet deposition, is this true?

Mulvihill: If you infuse platelet rich plasma for example with no red cells at all, you have a certain baseline retention, you do not have no retention at all on what is an activating artificial surface. On a collagen surface for instance, platelets will adhere, but from this baseline point adhesion increases with haematocrit up to about 35–40% red cell content and then you find there is no further effect. This has been shown in our system. One of the earlier tests we did to validate the system was to try to reproduce the experiments of others in relation to red blood cells and we found the same results.

Wautier: Do you think that the only role of red cells is to push platelets or is there something released from red cells that interacts with platelets?

Mulvihill: This is a point which has been greatly discussed: do red cells release ADP with stress and physical damage? I do not think the situation is entirely clear at the moment as to whether it is largely a physical or a

Y. F. Missirlis and J.-L. Wautier (eds.), The Role of Platelets in Blood-Biomaterial Interactions, 123–135.

haemodynamic effect. I would say that the most important factor is probably haemodynamic, but certainly under high stress and with turbulence as in an extracorporeal system, red cells may be damaged and release ADP. I think Mr Hansen may have practical experience on this point. Is there a real effect?

Hanson: We have not looked for a chemical effect of red cells on platelets but have studied the role of haematocrit on platelet thrombus formation. In these studies we measured platelet deposition from non-anticoagulated blood for periods up to 1 hour, a period longer than that usually reported in experimental studies. While there is probably a positive relationship between haematocrit and platelet deposition at low haematocrit, for haematocrit values between 20 and 55 we saw just the reverse since increasing the haematocrit in this range actually impaired platelet deposition. These studies suggest that the role of haematocrit may be more complicated than we appreciate based on earlier work.

Mulvihill: Let's go back to when you were observing decreases at higher red cell content and the effect of blood viscosity. Theoretically, excluding red cell effects, when you increase the viscosity of the blood you should impede the diffusion and transport of platelets.

Hanson: That could be a partial explanation.

Wautier: In the extracorporeal circulation the destruction of red cells result in haemolysis or fragmentation of the red cells, does this affect platelet function?

Davies: I think Steve Hanson said really what's known. My understanding is that nobody is very sure what the haemostatic effects of red cell lysates are, because there are some studies that show that red cells have got procoagulants in them and other studies that have failed to suppost that view.

Missirlis: I think also van Aken has reported that red cells can bind prostacyclin and the amount of binding depends on the shear forces that have been generated on the red cells. Coming back to the previous question, there have been studies by Goldsmith, and MacIntyre, and Scalak on the fluid mechanics around the rotating red cells. They have shown that local secondary flows might extend, so to speak, the diffusion of platelets to a greater extent, so that would make them to come into contact with the surface much faster. Also Sutera's group have measured the amount of ADP released by sublytic stress on the red cells and they saw a linear increase of adenosine being released from red cells. Of course in many experiments one must be very careful to define all the parameters that he used in this *in vitro* system to see whether artefacts are important or not, and one of my points when I presented my talk this morning was how other laboratories could duplicate *in vitro* studies. It seems that there is a problem there because the conditions are not defined clearly in most in-vitro experiments, that was ther point that I wish to make. And if I may ask a question – what is the role of the cytoskeleton on the mechanical properties of the platelets? Did I understand correctly that the uraemic platelets have no cytoskeleton?

Ordinas: Platelets are very similar to smooth muscle cells. The contents of actin and myosin are similar to those in platelet cytoskeletons. So, after a signal reaches the membrane a series of events develops leading to the assembly of the cytoskeleton. This assembly is followed by an internal contraction which is the same in both platelets and smooth muscle cells. I think that the cytoskeleton in platelets is like our skelton which facilitates movement which in platelets would be spreading and relates with the environment or with other cells in the case of platelets.

Missirlis: Does the cytoskeleton, then, provides a structural support when a platelet has to spread on a surface?

Ordinas: I think that the most important function of platelets is to have this ability.

Wautier: If I recall cytoskeleton in platelets is composed of two networks. One which is just under the membrane linked to the glycoprotein or the protein which is mostly responsible for the shape. There is another cytoskeleton which is in the center of the cell and is responsible for the extension of granules.

Davies: If we inhibit thrombin generation, do we need to do anything more to ensure adequate haemostasis in the patient? You spoke this morning about some studies in which you used activated protein C instead of a more conventional anticoagulant. To me that begged the question whether there is some inherent benefit in trying to switch off the coagulation mechanism at an earlier stage, rather than blocking thrombin.

Hanson: Our studies suggest that this may be the case. In primates, all direct antithrombins seem to produce significant bleeding at doses that are antithrombotic. Antithrombotic doses of activated protein C, which inactivates factors Va and VIIIa, or of agents which block factor Xa, produce considerably less bleeding. Therefore, the strategy of blocking earlier stages of the coagulation cascade may be a good one.

Davies: I have a simple-minded conception that effective antithrombotic treatments induce bleeding, and I also have difficulty with the idea that you can inhibit the coagulation mechanism at an earlier stage without having the same effect on bleeding.

Hanson: This raises the question of what constitutes significant clinical bleeding. We generally measure the bleeding time, which reflects small vessel or capillary bleeding from a superficial skin incision. However, this measurement does not necessarily predict surgical bleeding, joint bleeding, cerebral haemorrhage, hematoma formation, etc.

Davies: I think most people who have worked in clinical studies with platelets have taken the bleeding time as being a fairly specific indication of platelet function. We base that, I would guess, partly on the often quoted paper of Harker from the early 1970's showing that between 10–100,000 platelets per microlitre there was an almost linear correlation between platelet number and bleeding time. There are also observations that haemophilics have normal bleeding time. But the data that's coming through with the newer antithrombins would suggest that thrombin has a major influence on bleeding time and I find these thoughts difficult to reconcile.

Hanson: I don't have a problem accepting that thrombin may be the key activator of platelets *in vivo*, or that the bleeding time is a measure of platelet function. However, there is some controversy over whether the bleeding time can predict significant clinical bleeding. My view based on our animal studies is that very long bleeding times, say in excess of 30 minutes, do indicate a severe bleeding tendency and would, for example, predict increased surgical blood loss although more moderate prolongations of the bleeding time could be of little clinical consequence.

Davies: Do you have any thoughts, Jean-Luc, about bleeding time?

Wautier: Well I think that bleeding time is always difficult to perform.

Davies: But that's true in general. I don't think anyone knows how to predict which patient will bleed after cardiac bypass or which patients will bleed after straightforward surgical procedures, because surgical bleeding is a complex of many different technical factors, and factors in the patient. We know that some patients with haemostatic problems before surgery, are obviously at greater risk of bleeding in any of the procedures that we're talking about, but in patients who appear to have a normal haemostatic mechanism, I don't think anyone can predict which of those patients are liable to bleed.

Wautier: We have to take into account the fact that we add heparin to this system and we know that heparin could induce thrombocytopenia.

Mulvihill: With regard to the inhibition of thrombin earlier in the coagulation cascade, this would tie in with the use of low molecular weight heparinoids which is now fairly well established in preference to standard heparin. These compounds produce a sufficient anticoagulant effect without significant clinical bleeding or the large increase in bleeding time caused by heparin. It is now almost standard practice that people prefer the low molecular weight heparin fragments.

Davies: I'm not sure that I would altogether agree with that. I don't think the literature supports the view that the semi-synthetic and low molecular weight heparins cause less bleeding. Does anybody have any last thoughts about bypass?

Mulvihill: I would like to ask a question. I do not know whether people here have had any experience in modification of the surface itself, although I know that some Japanese groups in particular have tried to couple PGI2 or PGE1 to this kind of synthetic surface. Has anyone actually tested modified surfaces in connection with local inhibition of platelet deposition and activation, in other words not trying to infuse a product locally but to graft or link it to the surface itself in some way? Or is it a question of finance and are these surfaces likely to be highly expensive to produce? I myself have no personal experience of this approach but it is an interesting point.

Lemm: It is a topic for tomorrow morning, we will discuss it tomorrow morning.

Ordinas: I would just like to make a comment about bleeding in surgical procedures with extracorporeal circulation. I think that this problem has been drastically reduced over the past years, probably because of improvement in surgical techniques and also most of the procedures are no longer than one hour and a half. On the other hand, recently in cases in which the length of the procedure has been longer the use of a aprotinin, an inhibitor of fibrinolysis, has shown a reduction in bleeding.

Davies: There have been quite a number of groups who have shown that use a aprotinin significantly reduces blood loss, and most cardiothoracic surgeons now use it routinely. Quite how it works is still not absolutely certain, because the original studies suggested that it worked by preventing destruction of the platelet glycoprotein 1b and not all the groups using aprotinin have been able to confirm this. So, whether aprotinin works merely by preventing proteolytic cleavage of bits of platelets I think is open to question.

Perhaps I could start us off on the third of the topics, "Are antithrombotic peptides and monoclonal antiplatelet antibodies really new therapeutic agents". Clearly this is potentially a very big topic as well, depending on how far our collective knowledge stretches. Steve, again you probably have more experience than any of us, certainly a lot more practical experience than I do of the use of some of these new peptides. Can you take the discussion forward?

Hanson: Yes. This field was given great impetus by Barry Coller who developed antibody 7E3 against the platelet glycoprotein IIb/IIIa complex. In an elegant series of studies in dogs, monkeys, and then in humans, he showed that this antibody prevents fibrinogen binding to platelets, blocks platelet aggregation *ex vivo*, and inhibits thrombus formation *in vivo*. This antibody has gone into clinical trials, and may prevent rethrombosis following thrombolytic therapy. As a consequence of these studies a number of pharmaceutical companies are developing low molecular weight peptides containing an RGD (Arg-Gly-Asp) or similar sequences which, like antibody 7E3, specifically bind to GP IIb/IIIa and block its function. The thought is that these peptides will be less immunogenic than antibodies. They may also be safer since they have very short half-lives *in vivo*, and hence if the peptide infusion is stopped platelet function returns to normal within minutes to hours. With antibodies, which may circulate for many hours or days, there may be no antidote except to transfuse fresh platelets. For these reasons, the peptides are also in clinical trials; however, since they are given by continuous infusion they may be appropriate only for short-term indications like acute myocardial infarction, unstable angina, and to prevent reocclusion following angioplasty or thrombolytic therapy.

I suspect we will see limited application of antibodies like 7E3, but within several years very good peptides will be available which may become the preferred form of antiplatelet therapy. We have done a number of animal studies and find that the peptides also produce less bleeding than antibodies, when measured in terms of the bleeding time. This may be due to a faster off-rate of peptides vs antibodies, resulting in a more rapid restoration of platelet function when platelet plugs begin to form in the microcirculation. So, my view is that we are likely to see important clinical applications, particularly for the peptides. The next advance would be the development of stable organic inhibitors of GP IIb/IIIa which could be given orally. Although we have not worked with orally active agents, they are under development and, theoretically at least, would seem quite promising.

Davies: Chiara, you touched a little this morning on how the RGD peptides could be washed off the receptor. Do you know if there's any other data that would support the point that Steve's just made about how the reversal effect may be because the peptides come off again?

Kieffer: Yes, this morning we have discussed the results by DU and coworkers about RGD peptides as potential GPIIb-IIIa agonists. These results suggest that RGD peptides can function not only as GPIIb-IIIa inhibitors, but also as receptor agonists, however only in some very artificial experimental conditions. What DU and coworkers have shown is the following: An RGD peptide that binds to GPIIb-IIIa induces conformational changes of the receptor similar to those observed with fibrinogen: the peptide opens the receptor which exposes new high affinity binding sites for fibrinogen. If the peptide is eliminated through a washing procedure,then the receptor will close again. However, if the receptor is stabilized artificially in its open conformation by formaldehyde, and the peptide eliminated, then fibrinogen can bind. This experiment is intellectually very important and provides new information on GPIIb-IIIa, but the agonistic effect of the RGD peptide does not occur *in vivo*.

Davies: But it suggests as though something analogous might be.

Kieffer: The question is whether RGC, by interacting with GPIIb-IIIa does generate intracellular signals similar to those observed with fibrinogen.

Hanson: That doesn't seem to be the case. We've studied a variety of RGD peptides *in vivo* and they generally inhibit platelets and don't activate them. On the other hand, if you infuse certain antibodies, such as the anti-ligand induced binding site antibodies (anti-LIBS), you may see immediate and profound thrombocytopenia, probably because the antibody locks GP IIb/IIIa in a conformation that can bind fibrinogen which then may lead to platelet aggregation. In early studies antibody 7E3 also caused some drop in platelet count in patients. Subsequently, we've looked at an antibody against GP Ib in animals and this antibody produced severe thrombocytopenia by mechanisms that we don't understand, but which could involve signal transduction or receptor clustering. Thus, thrombocytopenia may be of concern with the use of antibodies, but perhaps not peptides, against platelet receptors.

I understand that with a humanized Fab fragment of 7E3 the problem of thrombocytopenia is largely eliminated.

Davies: Could we briefly consider the increasing tendency of drug companies and indeed academic institutions to patent their findings and treat them with exaggerated secrecy-how patentable, and how difficult to produce, are variants on RGD peptides. If such peptides cannot be protected, then organisations may decline to make them.

Hanson: I suspect that there are several patent positions for RGD and related peptides which are very strong, particularly since the companies with active programs include Merck, Genentech, Hoffman-LaRoche, and other large concerns.

Davies: Yes, its obviously a difficult topic but you've said enough to indicate that there would be plenty of ways in which more than one organisation could get into this game and potentially defend its position.

Wautier: To my knowledge the use of antibodies anti GPIIb/IIIa complex are effective for a very short period of time and you cannot used them for a long time. The injection of antibodies reduced the incidence of mistake angina. It is good at the time that you inject the antibodies, but afterwards when you need a second treatment, you cannot used the antibodies. One other point – antibodies are the same as peptides. The peptides has a very short half-life in the blood so it seems to be difficult at the present time to have drugs which have a short half-life to be used, or it will be very expensive treatment. Investigations now are trying to design drugs which are similar to the peptides instead of using peptides. So I am not sure there is a great future for the peptides. The other difficulty with the peptides which are like RGD peptides is that they are so ubiquitous that they can have so many side effects. Some of them were mentioned by Juliette this morning – the side effect on the endothelial cells and possibility on other cells – What could be also the effect of this peptide on the immune system? All these things as far as I know have been studied in *in vitro* system but what happens in the complete human system?

Mulvihill: With regard to effects on endothelial and other cells, I think at the moment we are at the stage of *in vitro* trials. These seem promising, but animal studies will certainly be required and eventually clinical trials, as experiments have as yet been largely limited to *in vitro* assays. Such experiments have been performed in connection with the detachment of endothelial cells by RGD peptides. One possible way around this problem could lie in the development by some groups of what you might call a complex peptide which shows RGD binding but also binding to the dodecapeptide sequence of the fibrinogen gamma chain. The resulting peptide is more specifically anti-fibrinogen rather than active against a wide range of adhesive proteins.

Kieffer: Yes, I think the second generation peptides will be receptor specific. I mean everybody's looking for this receptor specific. The first generation are RGD peptides or analogues, and now second generation peptides will be receptor specific peptides.

Hanson: Many peptides have been screened against other integrin receptors such as the vitronectin or fibronectin receptor, so that presently available peptides are in fact highly specific for GP IIb/IIIa and show little activity towards these other integrins.

Davies: I'd like to pick up a point you made, Jean-Luc, because I wouldn't necessarily agree with you that in the present context a short half-life is a disadvantage. Whereas clearly a short half-life is a disadvantage for systemic antithrombotic therapy, if you're trying to prevent platelet deposition on extracorporeal circuits then a short half-life is a positive advantage, because you cut down on "contamination" of the patient by the agent you've chosen to prevent blood reactions with the circuitry. So, for example, during use of prostacyclin in extracorporeal circuits short half- life is a positive advantage, rather than the reverse. So I would see that the potential field for agents of this type would be in reducing haemostatic reactions with extracorporeal circuitry. The question that concerns me is whether there is a clinical need for that, because of the advances in the design of the circuits that we have already talked about.

Wautier: For the first point, I think to have a short half-life is not a big problem except when you need a large amount of the product and it is very expensive. So the limitation is the price, it's not the fact that the product has a short half-life – it is the price of your treatment. But I think that probably the future in which we can be most optimistic is to have specific peptide or peptide analogues which can be specific for receptors. And I will probably be more happy to have this type of new products in the future than to have the real peptides. We are very happy with aspirin treatment but we know also that the aspirin has no effect on clinical situations like reocclusion after thrombolysis or restenosis after angioplasty and that all the treatment we have at the present time have no efficacy in this condition.

Davies: Those are where the clinical problems are, but they're a bit outside the field of this meeting. Clearly a potential target for which most clinicians want effective drugs is reocclusion in the coronary arteries. But in relation to blood reactions with artificial materials, is that such a big problem that we need to develop new agents?

Wautier: It depends, when you are looking at the thrombosis of articiifial graft and that's a major problem.

Hanson: There is another biomaterials application that is relevant to this discussion – that of the coronary endovascular stent. Following placement of these metallic devices patients commonly receive agressive antithrombotic therapy with heparin, coumadin, aspirin, dipyridamole, and dextran. Despite serious bleeding in about 30% of cases, approximately 5% of these stents undergo short-term occlusion. So here is an instance where a safe but effective therapy, perhaps an RGD peptide, could markedly expand the use of these devices which address a very important clinical problem.

Missirlis: Can I ask a question to the medical people? If you have a dialysis system, and you have heparin for anticoagulation, would you like to see a filter put after the dialysis system, where you have a resin to pick up heparin before it returns to the patient? Would that help avoid the bleeding problems? I mean you have to use heparin, or you are using heparin now, if somebody develops a polymer that could bind covalently heparin as soon as it comes out of the dialysis system, would you be happy with such a system?

Wautier: Well I think probably we would be happy with the system in which you have an anticoagulant or the antithrombotic product at the beginning that could be removed. Yes, I am not sure that we are very satisfied with it. I think heparin is one of the most usually but we know all the limitations of heparin, ie heparin is not good for platelets, heparin is not good for leukocytes, heparin also has some side effects. So heparin is not the answer by itself. We will be happy with such a system where you just put at the beginning of the extrapolysis systel the ideal antithrombotic products and you remove it at the end but just heparin itself, I think that's not the situation.

Hanson: I have one concern about regional anticoagulation – that is when you administer an agent at the device inlet and remove it at the outlet. There is still a region at the beginning of the circuit that may receive no treatment at all. Without some systemic anticoagulation you may have problems with the needles or cannulas used for blood access.

Davies: Almost certainly you will. That picks up a point in relation to the comment you made, Jean Luc, about intravascular grafts. As I understand it, intravascular grafts, whatever you make them of, stay more-or-less patent if they heve an internal, lumenal, diameter of larger than 8 mm. Smaller calibre grafts, particularly in the lower leg run into problems with reocclusion. That could be due to shear stress activation of platelet and under those circumstances, would an antithrombin be effective or would it be better to use an RGD against GpIIb/IIIa? what sort of compound will work under these circumstances?

Hanson: We have tried both, with encouraging results. When we placed 4 mm i.d. clinical grafts in primates, a single bolus injection of monoclonal antibody against GP IIb/IIIa markedly reduced acute thrombus formation and increased long-term patency rates. Since the antibody only circulated for about 48 hours, this result suggests that the early platelet reactions may be an important determinant of long-term outcomes. Similarly, when preclotted grafts are exposed directly, under static flow conditions *in vivo*, to potent antithrombins for even short time periods such as 15 minutes, these antithrombins can abolish the capacity of the graft to subsequently accumulate thrombus. This suggests that the thrombin present in these grafts, or in thrombus on the grafts, determines whether more thrombus accumulates and whether these grafts will occlude. Thus these newer therapies would seem promising to help prevent early graft occlusion. However, their affects on the secondary problem of late restenosis due to smooth muscle cell proliferation remain unknown.

Ordinas: In our Hospital the reocclusion of the bypass in patients after cardiovascular surgery have shown that the percentage of reocclusion in grafts of less than 1 1/2 mm after one month is 40%, while in grafts larger than 2 mm the percentage of reocclusion is 25%. I think that this information must be taken into account when developing biomaterial for this purpose.

Mulvihill: I would agree that it is the narrow vascular grafts which cause problems. A wide bore graft in the coronary circulatory system is at much lower risk for thrombosis, but the vascular surgeons nevertheless prefer to use a saphenous vein graft if possible. They use an artificial implant almost as a last resort knowing very well that they will have about a 40% reocclusion rate. I think that for artificial implants in this situation, something that could stop acute platelet deposition over a 24–48 hr period might not solve the whole problem but would certainly be a start. This relates to earlier work by Mustard and his group, who showed that if you could prevent the initial platelet deposition following removal of the endothelium, after about 48 hr the exposed surface became less thrombogenic and there was much less platelet deposition. Thus it seemed even in these early experiments that it was the initial period that was critical. If you could stop the process early on, later you had less serious problems, so an inhibitor with a short half-life could in fact be of great value. One further comment, you mentioned that in dialysis systems you have platelet activation before heparin and we have certainly experienced this in our *ex vivo* tests. We use heparin injection just after the point of venous access and therefore the needle and a very short section of synthetic tubing are exposed to the blood before heparin injection. If we use a wide bore needle we have very few problems, but at one stage we tried a finer needle and found that about one in three would completely occlude. Hence there is activation in the absence of heparin at the point of needle insertion. In dialysis patients, if you remove the heparin after the dialysis module, then this will not be returned to the circulation system and you might therefore have to use more heparin on the in-line because it is not recirculated. Over a period of 3 hr with systemic heparinisation of the patient, heparin will be re-used. If at each passage through the dialyser you inject it and then remove it – is this really of great value? Particularly as I am not aware that bleeding is a problem in routine dialysis, or rarely, perhaps certain patients who have haemostatic problems. In general, for uraemic patients without other haemostatic problems, the low amounts of heparin employed for dialysis do not present many problems.

Missirlis: But what I understand from Jean-Luc is that the less heparin you have in the systemic circulation, the better it is, is that true?

Mulvihill: Yes.

Davies: I am not sure how much further we can take it. I would be interested to know what you feel is going to be the front runner. We've talked mainly about RGD peptides and have not talked much about PPACK(D-Phe-Pro-ArgCH_2Cl) and its variants.

Hanson: I believe both newer antiplatelet agents and antithrombins will be used. Since PPACK is likely to be toxic, I doubt if it will be used in man. Hirudin may, depending on its cost, safety threshold, and antigenicity. Hirudin analogs, such as hirulog, are likely to be used and particularly in venous thrombosis and perhaps in heparin-induced thrombocytopenia. Since we do not yet have oral agents of these types, both the new antithrombins and RGD-type peptides will probably be used to prevent short-term vessel occlusion in a number of settings.

Davies: Yes, I think hirudin is one of the most promising. If it could be marketed at a price that is competitive with heparin, it gives the advantage of a linear dose-response effect on coagulation tests. Its big disadvantage, as we talked about this morning, is that so far there is not a specific inhibitor of hirudin activity, but it would be an easier compound to work with. It might, of course, have some unforeseen side-effects in long-term use as heparin has turned out to have. But in practice, the problems with heparim of thrombocytopenia, and osteoporosis, and hair loss and so on, are not widely seen, unless you have used heparin for extended periods of time.

Missirlis: Can I ask again one question? If you put an arterial graft into the body is it better to, for example, bind hirudin or albumin or heparin onto it and preserve its function rather than give it systemically?

Hanson: The concept of binding antithrombotics has been around a long time, notably the binding of heparin. It could be argued that heparin binding to surfaces could actually be detrimental, since the surface might then act as a sink for thrombin thereby increasing its local concentration. Also, when surfaces are modified in this way it is difficult to know whether an observed benefit is due to a specific drug action, or simply to the change in surface physicochemical properties, effects on protein adsorption, etc. I have yet to see convincing data that surface-immobilized drugs provide a long-term benefit, although a short-term benefit with devices like dialyzers and catheters may be achieved, particularly if the drug elutes. With immobilized small molecules, there are questions of drug conformational alterations and the ability of tethered agents to effectively interact with target receptors, enzymes, etc. For long-term applications, there are also questions of immobilized drug degradation and masking by deposited blood elements.

Lemm: I have only one question because I am not familiar with this topic but aprotinin is also a peptide. It was not yet mentioned, do you have experience with it?

Davies: Perhaps we have not talked about it much because it is not an antithrombin and it is not, as far as we know, a platelet inhibitor. It was originally used for the treatment of pancreatitis, althrough I think there is little evidence that even in pancreatitis it is effective. Now it is enjoying a second life as a blood sparing agent in cardiopulmonary bypass. My reading of the literature is that I do not think we are yet certain how it works, although probably it works as a fibrinolytic inhibitor.

Wautier: We know that aprotinin is also acting on the coagulation, on the fibrinolytic, and complement system. Aprotinin is a drug which is acting at different levels so its really difficult just to know what is the final effect of all these actions on the coagulation and on the platelet function. We know that platelet functions are slightly modifed by aprotinin indirectly by it could modified plasmatic factor that could affect platelet function. I am not happy myself by putting anticoagulant like heparin on biomaterial which will be used as graft for the reason that we need cells on this graft at one end and if we avoid what is the first step the fibrin-fibrinogen formation which is one of the best conditions to permit the cells to adhere and grow on the graft, it is bad. So I will be happy just to have one line of fibrin not a big thrombus, but one line of fibrin or one line of platelets which avoids the construction of big thrombus and after that the cells can migrate into the graft. Then it can work properly.

Missirlis: Even for small diameter vessels? Because for large diameters what you said is working, is patent, but for a size of 1.5 mm in diameter do you need a layer of cells and proteins to develop onto the grafts?

Wautier: If you don't have the cells at the beginning in, you will have afterwards around and they will reject all the material so you can have benefit in the first 2 or 3 days and in the next weeks a disaster. The better is probably to have something which is the most similar to what is in the subendothelial matrix. Some surgeons are telling that they use now graft for vessel transplantation. They are using vessels as they are using heart or liver to transplant from one patient to another. They say that they have big troubles when they use the vessel which has just been taken from the donor, but when they keep it for 1–2 days in bad conditions for biologists in their poor conservative medium they have better results in transplantation. This probably means that most of the cells which are in the vessel have been completely destroyed and are no longer there. They have a thrombogenic surface – exactly what we use as perfect thrombogenic surface and they say it works better – I don't know if this is true but that's the experiments. We know also that in some conditions when you have one line of platelets which have adhered to the subendothelium you don't have a big thrombus and this line of platelets seems to be non-reactive for a second activation of platelets, that could be an appropriate reaction of the body. Trying to mimic some of the bad way we have the opposite result that we are expecting.

11. Platelet and biomaterials, extracorporeal circulation and implanted materials

Lemm: In our context biomaterials are understood as synthetic polymers which will contact blood. Apart from this another large group of biomaterials are applied as bone or dental materials. In modern medicine such materials are used in large quantities: 6.5 million dialysers, 70 000 heart valves a year in Europe. One single German company produces between 1000 and 2000 km of medical grade PVC tubings. Despite the economic importance of such devices not all details of the blood-material-interaction are known. Thrombus formation on an artificial surface is still an unsolved problem. The perfect non-thrombogenic surface does not yet exist. Apart from thrombocytes a variety of blood proteins are involved in the genesis of thrombus formation.

During this morning session I would like to elaborate some suggestions how to design an improved hemocompatible surface for different applications.

The so-called initial event is briefly described by the Lyman hypothesis: a high affinity of an artificial surface to albumin indicates good hemocompatibility, while on the other side a preference for fibrinogen points to a poor thromboresistance. Controversially discussed are the hypotheses of hydrophilic/hydrophobic surfaces and negatively/positively charged interfaces.

I would suggest to start with the problem of blood-material-interaction. What do you think is really the initial step, is it protein adsorption or is it platelet adhesion?

Hanson: It is generally thought that protein adsorption occurs first, simply because proteins are smaller than cells, and therefore diffuse faster and reach the surface more quickly. Blood proteins may adsorb to every surface studied including hydrophobic surfaces like Teflon and hydrophilic polymers such as the highly hydrated hydrogels. Thus, my understanding is that proteins adsorb first, and that these proteins subsequently mediate adhesion of platelets and other cells.

Mulvihill: This is the general assumption. Certainly if you analyse any of these surfaces after blood contact, in my experience you never find protein not to be there, whether or not blood cells come afterwards, which is generally accepted to be the case.

Wautier: Does that mean that because it is generally accepted that it's true?

Y. F. Missirlis and J.-L. Wautier (eds.), The Role of Platelets in Blood-Biomaterial Interactions, 137–151.

Mulvihill: Theoretically it follows.

Hanson: Experimentally as well, since all surfaces seem to adsorb proteins.

Wautier: I think I agree that the surface can attract protein. That's most of the cases. But if I think very simply I think it should be similar at what it happens if you stop bleeding and everything is coming at the same time, the proteins are interacting with the subendothelial surfaces and the cells too. So I don't see any reason why it should be different when you have an artificial surface. My guess is that at the same time you have the activation of the platelets, leucocyte, that you have some collision with the red cells, and that all sorts of plasma proteins are sticking and the configuration is modified by the hemocompatible surface. I would say it's always difficult to tell what comes first, I would prefer to think that everything is starting at the same time but with different kinetics.

Mulvihill: I think the time delays must be very short, a matter of fractions of a second between protein and cellular deposition. Then of course it is also a dynamic surface. There are groups who have demonstrated with radiolabelled proteins, antibodies and other techniques that there is protein exchange and change of conformation. The reactivity towards antibodies will change. It is also possible with leucocytes that you could have protein lysis on the surface under cells which perhaps contact and are then removed. The nature of the proteins underneath could be altered as a result.

Wautier: I have a question for people who are more familiar than me with that. Do we know if there is exchange of proteins? We know that in some systems you have to let proteins for 24 hr with surface in the system to be sure that there is very little detachment of the protein from the plastic surface. Do we know that there is some exchange? That some proteins come first and detach from the surface and other proteins come second and there is some exchange of proteins on the biocompatible surface?

Mulvihill: Well, there is the well known Vroman effect, that generally the smaller protein molecules adsorb first. You find on a surface in contact with plasma a mixture of albumin, fibrinogen, fibronectin, immunoglobulins and other less abundant proteins, which will tend to be replaced later by predominantly fibrinogen and then at a further stage HMWK and even larger molecules. But this again depends on the kind of surface. The Vroman effect has been found to be true for hydrophilic surfaces, whereas on hydrophobic materials you do not always find the same result. So it must depend on the primary interaction whether exchange takes place or not.

Missirlis: However the Vroman effect has not been proven conclusively under flow conditions. It's considered mostly for static conditions. However, again, the most prevalent idea now is that there is a continuous exchange and it has to do also with the type of surface. Now many people produce surfaces with different microdomains, different structures, different properties, so to speak. And so what the proteins see isn't the same all over the surface. And the idea of conformational changes of those proteins when they attach themselves or they come within the boundary layer where they are ready to attach to the surface it is something that, to my opinion, is not clear yet, because you measure the end effect. You don't have probes to see what happens when the protein comes there. You see it after it has reached the place. And most of the time they are radio labeled, and then how different is the hot from the cold protein?

Hanson: There is certainly a large literature on this subject. The time course of adsorption of different proteins depends strongly of the nature of the substrate surface. Once adsorbed, proteins may undergo a variety of conformational alterations and additional binding interactions as shown with radiolabelled proteins, as well as by changes in elutability, for example by SDS, and also by changes in antigenicity as detected with various antibodies. So, it's a very complex dynamic process that is not well understood at the present time.

One important question is why platelets recognize surface adsorbed fibrinogen and not soluble fibrinogen. If fibrinogen is really the important adhesive glycoprotein for platelets, how does its binding to surfaces support subsequent platelet reactions.

Kieffer: We have to consider that immobilized fibrinogen is structurally and antigenically different from soluble fibrinogen. Indeed, there are monoclonal antibodies available today that interact with immobilized but not with soluble fibrinogen. One of these monoclonal antibodies identifies an epitope located on the C-terminal part of the fibrinogen γ chain, about 20 amino acids apart from the dodecapeptide site, suggesting that the C-terminus of the γ chain undergoes a conformational change and becomes accessible to the monoclonal antibody when fibrinogen is bound to a surface.

Missirlis: Then the question arises: if a fibrinogen molecule which has attached itself and changed its conformation on the surface, and maybe has been denatured, what happens after it is replaced by IgG, for example, does it regain its original properties?

Kieffer: I have no experience in that field. I don't know.

Mulvihill: In fact IgG is also fairly reactive towards platelets, especially as platelets have a receptor for the Fc fragment of IgG. If you imagine a surface bearing IgG adsorbed in a conformation with the Fc region directed out towards the contacting plasma medium, then platelets will react with this surface. On the other hand, if you have a surface which tends to adsorb IgG with the Fc region down towards the surface, these binding sites will not be exposed. Hence IgG is not necessarily less thrombogenic than fibrinogen. Depending on the surface, it can be highly reactive too.

Kieffer: Fibrinogen might function in a similar way as vWF. The soluble plasma vWF does not bind to platelets. Only vWF that has undergone conformational changes-by binding to the subendothelial matrix-mediates platelet adhesion through the GPIb-IX complex.

Similarly, soluble fibrinogen cannot interact with resting platelets. But once it is bound to a surface it promotes resting platelet adhesion.

Wautier: There is a similar situation for fibronectin and leucocytes. The fibronectin which is in solution has not the same configuration as fibronectin which is attached to a surface. Fibronectin attached to a surface is better attractant for monocyte and polymorphonuclear which have a specific receptor for fibronectin and it has been very well demonstrated by electron microscopy of the molecule itself that we can see there is change in the conformation of the molecule. And I don't think we have to speak about denaturation, is not denaturation it's something different.

Missirlis: But if I understood it correctly you have the flowing blood, where a fibrinogen molecule may come into collision with a platelet and they will not react. What happens then when the fibrinogen molecule sticks onto a surface and a platelet comes onto it? Does it react? I mean as I understood from what you said yesterday there are 50,000 receptors around the platelets, so as I can see it is that everywhere there is a receptor to attach to fibrinogen. What makes it not an effective attachment during flow in normal blood and this is not the case when the fibrinogen molecule is sticking onto a surface.

Davies: You don't necessarily have to postulate that the protein is reacting with the resting platelet because in an intact circulation, I can not conceive how you can put in any kind of vascular prosthesis without causing shear-stress to the platelets. There is a lot of evidence that in shear fields platelets become activated. Now you can almost certainly-although it cannot be proved in the intact animal-but you can almost certainly get platelet microaggregates formed in shear fields, and presumably under those circumstances platelets become activated and react with fibrinogen in the fluid phase.

So I don't think that you necessarily need to say that fibrinogen when it's surface bound, even if it's chemically different in its physicochemical characteristics, has to react with platelets in a different way. It may react in the same way but it may be the platelets that are activated.

Wautier: I think there is another point. Probably the affinity between the molecule and the cell is very different. That means that with a force which is smaller you can detach one from other. But when the affinity is higher you cannot detach one from the other. And when you look under microscope what the platelet is doing, most of the time a platelet is coming to stick to something that is going on and when it is the appropriate receptor, collagen or matrix proteins, platelets is stick and other platelets come and then the clot is becoming to grow so I think it just a difference in affinity between the protein and the platelets. That the affinity between the protein and the platelets, the affinity is becoming 1,000 higher so you cannot detach the one from the other.

Lemm: We observed another effect, which is difficult to explain. Hydrophobic surfaces, such as silicones, adsorb preferably fibrinogen. Fillers are added to regular silicones for a better mechanical stability. But only these silicones are rather thrombogenic; filler-free silicones adsorb fibrinogen as well but their thrombogenic properties are much better. What is the reason for this behaviour?

Mulvihill: We have had similar experience working with protein adsorption on dialyser membranes. Generally, fibrinogen adsorption increases platelet adhesion on all membranes but to a different extent according to the membrane surface. In the case of polyacrylonitrile, it seems to have a particularly bad effect and activates these membranes with respect to platelet adhesion more strongly than others. We thought it might be interesting to find out, possibly with monoclonal antibody probes, whether fibrinogen is adsorbed in a specific configuration on the membranes according to their chemical structure. This was one hypothesis we put forward to explain our results. There was an almost ten fold effect on platelet accumulation on polyacrylonitrile as compared to a two or three fold effect on polysulphone or cuprophan membranes. It would seem to depend on a specific characteristic interaction which puts a molecule in a certain conformation according to the surface where it is adsorbed.

Kieffer: That is certainly a reasonable hypothesis. I have a question: is fibrinogen the only major plasma protein that promotes the biomaterial/platelet interaction and is this interaction dependent on the platelet fibrinogen receptor GPIIb-IIIa, which is a member of the integrin family of cell adhesion receptors? Could other integrins of the platelet membrane also be involved? I think in particular of the fibronectin receptor. It has been reported that the fibronectin receptor can directly interact with a plastic surface in the absence of the ligand fibronectin and that cell adhesion to plastic is essentially mediated through the fibronectin receptor.

Hanson: It may not be entirely clear that fibrinogen is essential. Years ago we defibrinogenated animals with the snake venom Ancrod, which produces a total absence of detectable fibrinogen in clotting assays. However, platelet thrombi formed in a seemingly normal manner on artificial surfaces exposed to blood from these animals. This result doesn't preclude the importance of fibrinogen under normal circumstances since platelets may have released granular fibrinogen which was protected from the enzyme, and because it is only in the absence of available fibrinogen that the platelet reactions may be supported by other plasma glycoproteins such as von Willebrand factor. However, this result does suggest that the preadsorption of circulating clottable fibrinogen may not be required to initiate the process.

Davies: But that is difficult to interprete because ancrod clips the A-peptide from the amino terminal end of the molecule. As I understand it, that is not near the parts of the molecule that react with platelets.

Hanson: Ancrod produces a variety of fragments from the fibrinogen molecule which, although not clottable, could adsorb and support platelet adhesion. Thus while the experiment doesn't answer all questions, but it does raise some issues regarding the role of fibrinogen.

Davies: Yes, it certainly answers ther question whether you need clottable firbrinogen.

Wautier: We had the observation of a patient with afibrinogenemia and who developed an arterial thrombotic disorder with platelet aggregates in his legs so it seems that *in vivo* at least platelet aggregation can occur in absence of fibrinogen.

Hanson: Yes, that's been shown by others, too.

Wautier: Yes, but not in a test tube, in his own vessels.

Kieffer: I think they are competing ligands for the same receptor. So, if one competitor is absent, then the other one can interact with the receptor.

Wautier: Yes.

Mulvihill: There is also vWF which especially under high shear conditions has been shown to be involved in platelet spreading and stabilization of thrombi. If vWF is not present, these events are in fact impaired. Certainly there are competitive effects, as the RGD sequence is present on fibronectin, vWF and fibrinogen. Perhaps if one molecule, fibrinogen for instance, is absent then the others will compensate for this lack.

Wautier: But if you put the question another way, what is the best to have no protein on a surface or to have protein which is less reactive with the cells?

Lemm: We discussed this question three years ago. How should a surface be designed? Should it exhibit no affinity to any protein, and thus be proteinophobic? Or should the surface select specific proteins? An efficient technique in surgery in the pre-albuminisation of surfaces which will prevent platelet adhesion.

Mulvihill: On a practical basis, it is simple and highly effective.

Lemm: It is, yes.

Mulvihill: We certainly found this to be true in plasmapheresis circuits. In our patients, it seemed not to be a fibrinogen problem but more probably small aggregates of abnormal immunoglobulin molecules capable of forming immune complexes. This was the reason for which they were undergoing plasmapheresis therapy, to remove immune complexes and aggregated IgG. We encountered blockage of the plasmapheresis circuit with platelet-fibrin thrombi and the way to avoid this problem was to carry out albumin passivation of the entire circuit. This worked very well. In the filters, for example, when we looked at them with and without albumin treatment, one would be clean and the other red and clotted. These results would however raise one question: is it always fibrinogen? In this case we found not. Our patients had normal fibrinogen and it was the IgG which seemed to be causing problems.

Missirlis: However albumin may solve the problem for a short time. It may be replaced further on. But suppose a manufacturer gives us a new material to be tested whether it is better or worse from others in terms of thrombogenicity. What would be the relevant in-vitro tests to do it? If you put it in a circuit and you don't see any platelets adhere, is it a good test by itself? I think people do selective tests according to their ideas and I haven't seen in the literature a set of tests that, put together, would give an answer, more relevant to what would happen *in vivo*. So maybe we should discuss or decide what are the most relevant tests to do and combine them in order to give an answer.

Ordinas: This should be discussed later this afternoon but if you like it could be discussed now.

Davies: I am interested in what you said, Dr. Lemm, that if protein polymer chemists were given a brief, you thought with today's skills they could design a surface more-or-less with the properties requested. Why has nobody tried – or perhaps they have and I don't know – why has nobody tried to produce a surface that doesn't react with proteins, because it is a reasonable hypothesis that such surfaces would be less reactive than surfaces which react with proteins. We know that if you are going to pick a protein to make a surface less reactive there is a wealth of evidence that albumin is more-or-less nonreactive with platelets, though there is the problem of protein exchange with time. It seems to me that the idea that cells in a high flow situation will react with glass or plastic or other synthetic surface with a high affinity and without an intermediate protein is improbable. If you designed a surface that didn't react with protein, it may react to a very low level with circulating cells also.

Wautier: Can I just make a point. If we think that the endothelium is the best surface for hemocompatibility, when the endothelium is normal, what the endothelium is doing. It is doing a lot of things : it is secreting products which limit the activation of platelets, have receptors to limit the activation of coagulation, and also is secreting products that can destroy in a way or activate the fibrinolytic system. So it is always a dynamic condition. So if we try to reproduce something which its similar to endothelium we have to have not only a good surface, we have to add all these products at the same time to limit the coagulation, to dissolve the clot, when the clot is forming, and to limit the platelet activation. So we cannot have a surface without adding substances which will play the same role as the endothelium is doing.

Davies: But we must be light years away, technically, from being able to reproduce the biochemistry of endothelial cells. Because although we know thrombosis releases various things that can turn on endothelial cell release of tPA, and PGI_2, we don't know what the controlling mechanisms are *in vivo*. Nor do we know whether intermittent release of any of these substances is what gives an endothelial cell surface its lack of reactivity in the hemostatic mechanism. Although the experimental work is convincing, it is still speculative whether in the circulation it is surface glycosaminoglycans or thrombomodulin or other factors which inactivate thrombin. We don't really know, it seems to me, why the endothelial cell surface is non reactive to the haemostatic mechanism.

Ordinas: In patients with replacement of a heart valve or even in some other prosthesis the prosthesis itself becomes covered with endothelial cells and becomes like real endothelium and so biomaterials implanted in the human become like a real artery or real vein.

Davies: Correct me if I am wrong, but I thought that in humans, unlike some animals, endothelial cells would not grow in very far from the edge of a graft, and that if you seeded grafts with endothelial cells, you get growth of endothelium, but it wouldn't grow to confluence.

Wautier: I think it depends on the time you have to put this in the body. There are circulating endothelial cells and we don't knows, what are these circulating endothelial cells. Are they really detatched endothelial cells because they are dead or are they some cells that can regrow again. When you take the endothelial cells from the culture which are detatched and you put them in a new culture plate they grow again. So it doesn't mean because they are detatched and they are in the circulation that they are really dead cells. I'm not sure that the cell you see on a graft which has been in a patient for years it's almost covered everywhere with cells which have not exactly the same feature as endothelial cells but they may be fibroblasts.

Missirlis, Davies: They may be fibroblasts.

Wautier: I am not sure at all they are fibroblasts. You have to have the appropriate marker just to know what type of shells. Because if you put the cells in culture and you just add something they look like fibroblasts but they are not.

Missirlis: I think, at least the literature shows, that what Dr. Davies said is right, that at least in small diameter posthesis you have only in the anastomotic sides some endothelialization. But if you culture cells and you put them before implantation on the substrate you don't see afterwards only pseudoendothelial cells but also fibroblasts, smooth muscle cells are coming there, and some of them could produce materials that are thrombogenic. There are two lines, I think, in this area. One is to cover the surfaces with endothelial or endothelial – like cells.

Another one is to bind various molecules, either 2 types like the group of Feijen is doing: PGI_2 or albumin and heparin together with different ligands. John Brash in Canada is trying to put fibrinolytic molecules, not only urokinase but others as well, on to the polyurethanes he is producing. According to your suggestion, one should try to put not only anticoagulant but also fibrinolytic molecules on the surface hoping that they are viable at long times, forever, if possible. You know, this is a strategy, but I think again we don't see, at least, I haven't seen, how you can monitor this process, how you can say: well I put with this ligand a heparin molecule or PGI_2 and I know it is viable and it hasn't changed its properties. Because when I put it in an animal and I see some thrombi, I don't know where they have originated.

Davies: I think that although that is an approach worth exploring, in my opinion, it is an approach that is not going to work for the reason that I tried to outline before. The evidence is lacking that an intact endothelium in an undamaged circulation, is releasing these molecules into the circulation. I think the endothelium switches on thrombomodulin activity, releases tPA and releases PGI_2 when something happens. But if nothing has happened, I doubt whether this dynamic interaction with the blood is going on all the time. Moncada and Vane were the first to suggest that PGI_2 is a circulating hormone, and that endothelial cells secreted a little PGI_2 all the time, but the evidence for this is not there. And so I would come back to the point I was trying to make originally, that one area to look at would be to make a synthetic surface which doesn't react with plasma proteins. I suspect that when we understand how the endothelium works in the intact circulation, we will find that there is little continuous physico-chemical interaction between endothelial cells and the proteins in blood. We know that endothelial cells can react with a whole range of plasma proteins but the question is: do they react in the intact circulation? And I suspect that perhaps they don't.

Ordinas: I am not sure that I agree with you in what you said about the endothelium not continuously changing. You are thinking about producing a prosthesis tube through which the blood will flow. However, depending on the site of implantation of the prosthesis the mechanics and necessesities will vary since the hemodynamics may be completely different at each site the same as with endothelium damage which is generally found at the site of bifurcations. These sites are precisely where atherosclerotic lesions appear since the blood flow and thus the hemodynamics differ and there is continuous removal of endothelial cells. So to complement the discussion a little we are talking about new biomaterials in a tube and maybe they have nothing to do with other biomaterials required with this type of situation as with bifurcation and others which are completely different such as with a little patch put into the aorta in a patient after an aneurysm.

Wautier: I don't agree at all with Andrew Davies when he said that there is no evidence that there are secreted products from the endothelial cells. There is a lot of evidence. First that there is a basal secretion of PGI2. You can measure in some conditions. We know also that a very largely used test in clinics is that when we apply the venostasis you release TPA from the local vein so there is stimulation that makes TPA secretion. We have good evidence that when you are using a vein for coronary bypass instead of an artery the results are always much better with arteries than with veins and one thing proposed to explain the difference is that when you are using an artery the production of nitric oxide is higher and when you use a vein it is lower. So I think we have good evidence that there is an active process occuring at the endothelial cell level in the normal body.

Hanson: There is also evidence for *in vivo* modulation of coagulation reactions. For example, in normal individuals there are measurable levels of prothrombin fragment 1.2 and activated protein C. The continuous activation of protein C may be important since severe protein C deficiency is not compatible with life. So, there may always be a continuous basal coagulation process that is probably regulated by the endothelium.

Missirlis: I would also think that it would be quite improbable to have a system dormant for long times. And then suddenly something happens and it wakes up. I mean not only from the endothelial cells but from bone, from all types of organs. I think that there is a basal dynamic action all the time. But coming back to your question why don't people produce proteinophobic materials, well, at least all the materials that have been tested and we know of, adsorb proteins...

Lemm: Well, to a different degree.

Missirlis: Yes to a different degree, but they do adsorb. Theoretically even if you were able to produce in the lab a surface that is proteinophobic, when you come to manufacturing it there are so many other parameters, in the extrusion process or in other types of manufacturing your material, that is quite improbable that some molecules that would be there, either a lubricant, or the ethylenoxide, or some gas, or whatever you use in the production, is going to attract proteins. But even if you solve this problem, I think especially in arterial graft prosthesis the biggest problem is suturing. Because there you will create a surface which will attract all kinds of proteins and cells. So even if you have the best material, the problem is, at this tiny part which will be sutured or I don't know later on, maybe by lasers you can connect the living and the non living substance and then you create an endothelial surface there and so the blood doesn't see at all this interface. I think the biggest problem would be that small interface. And some studies indicate at least in the small diameter vasculature that they try to produce, that problems originate at that anastomotic surface.

Kieffer: Because it creates additional troubles.

Missirlis: Yes.

Davies: I obviously accept the point my colleagues make that there is a low background level of PGI_2 in urine, although the levels in plasma are undetectable with current methodology.

And the idea that the coagulation and the fibrinolytic systems are switched on all the time at a very low level is a concept 30–40 years old. Astrup proposed in the mid-1950s that fibrolysis was permanently switched-on at a low level. But these things are happening at a very low level indeed and maybe, for example, the tPA or PGI_2 that is released from endothelium is released only at those branching points that have been referred to, at which the endothelium is under stress. So, I am not saying that the endothelium has no interaction with the blood. Perhaps I am asking the question whether the interactions of which we are well aware are the main mechanism which prevents a resting endothelium reacting with blood components in a free flowing situation. If you calculate the amount of tPA or PGI_2 that is available on the surface of a large artery it's not sufficient to prevent most of the reactions that we are talking about. Most of the PGI_2 and the tPA is released into the microcirculation, because that's where the great bulk of the endothelium is. So, I am happy with the concept that most of these systems are there to deal with some changed circumstance, with some kind of vascular injury. I just speculate that perhaps we are oversimplifying things if we think that those systems are the main reason why the blood doesn't interact with the normal endothelium in a large blood vessel. If we knew more about what these processes are, we might be better at designing artificial materials.

If we can reject the idea of trying to design a surface which doesn't react with blood then we are left with trying to design a surface which preferentialy attracts those proteins that we think it ought to attract. There is not much doubt that the protein should be albumin. So the key question is how do you stop albumin from exhanging with other plasma proteins, and what is it about the surface that makes that happen.

Lemm: One approach is the immobilisation of receptors which bind specifically albumin in order to have a permanently stable albumin layer. Another approach is the extremely hydrophilic surface which does not adsorb proteins at all. A long time ago, Andrade published that water is the best biomaterial. Such hydrogels behave as good as the extremely hydrophobic surfaces.

Hanson: We have evaluated highly hydrated materials, so-called hydrogels containing 80–90% water which were based on acrylic and methacrylic polymers and copolymers. These surfaces did adsorb proteins and were thrombogenic by a mechanism involving the continuous formation and embolization of small platelet thrombi. Thus while these materials seemed less thromboadherent, since large thrombi were not seen, they nonetheless caused excessive consumption of platelets. The strategy of using highly hydrophilic surfaces may therefore have some limitations.

Cerletti: I have a question. Did anybody consider the possibility of stimulating adhesion of endothelial cells to the biomaterial *in vivo*? I know that in-vitro it has been tried.

Mulvihill: It is difficult to find a substrate to which endothelial cells will adhere and then grow and be viable. We have had a little experience in this field in trying to coat biomaterials with fibronectin, for instance, which is a well known concept. We also tried a simulation of the preclotting technique used to seed surgical implants, a mixture of fibrinogen and thrombin which would clot on the surface. Then we tried a biological glue, transglutine, which in fact worked well to attach the endothelial cells. However the problem seemed to be that in a static system you could get the cells to adhere and even grow to confluence but when you put the surface under flow conditions you tended to lose about 60% of the cells. Transglutine gave the most adherent surface. Fibronectin gave us, quite frankly, poor results and preclotting was not too bad. I think that the endothelium is such a complex system, to try to reproduce it chemically or physicochemically by binding PGI2, albumin-heparin or other molecules expressing particular aspects of endothelial activity is very difficult. The alternative is to try to obtain a viable endothelium which will do its normal job. In this case the trouble is to attach it, especially in humans. I would agree with Prof. Missirlis that normally you can get a confluent endothelium growing on prostheses in animals, as in baboons and certainly in dogs. In human beings, on the other hand, you may find a little ingrowth from the suture points at the two ends of the graft, but the middle section even after long periods, although sometimes apparently covered with cells, does not develop a viable and non thrombogenic endothelium.

Hanson: In some animals you do achieve complete coverage. In primates the cells migrate in from the cut ends of adjacent vessel to an extent greater than that seen in man, but may not proceed to complete graft coverage. Such grafts may remain indefinitely thrombogenic as shown by non-invasive platelet imaging of Dacron grafts as late as 10 years following implantation. More recently, Teflon grafts have also shown late platelet accumulations and thus may never heal completely. Only rarely has complete graft endothelialization been reported in man, and even in these instances there may be some questions of cell identification.

Missirlis: I have two questions here. One is: are all endothelial, arterial endothelial cells the same? I mean, if you take endothelial cells from, say, a large artery and from a small arteriole are they the same functionally? And the second is: has somebody studied the growth factors that an endothelial cell produces in order to go further? So why it so happens in humans that they grow a little bit and then they stop suddenly? Is it some mechanism that cannot produce the material to stick? Has somebody studied that?

Wautier: But I think the answer is simple and not that simple. The first simple thing to say is that the endothelial cells are different in the veins from the arteries, and they are different in the big vessel and the small vessel, and the post-capillary endothelial cells are different too, but they have the potential to be stimulated and to become not that different. So, they are different in the normal condition. But ig you look at some receptors which are nonexpressed on cells in large arteries they can be expressed in some pathological condition or when they have been simulated by some cytokines. So, in normal condition they are different but you can make them similar in stress condition. That's the first point.

The second point is when, you know that the replacement of endothelial cells in normal body is very low, it's between months and years. So in some vessels the turnover is very low. When you culture endothelial cells in presence of growth factor for months, you find that after several divisions the endothelial cells become different. They lose after some divisions their initial properties and in terms of their non-thrombogenicity and production of different factors. For human endothelial cells after 12 passages they stop dividing. They are still endothelial cells, they are still living cells, but they are unable to divide again. This observation could fit with the theory that the number of divisions of a cell is limited.

Missirlis: Genetically?

Wautier: Genetically, it depends on the cell and there is great theory that say that the life, our life expectancy is depending upon the number of division a cell is able to make. If we damage endothelial cells at one point they can be replaced the first time but if we smoke as my good friend Danny does, you damage the endothelial cells. The damaged cell is a good cell but after that is becoming less good and its capacity of proliferation is reduced even in presence of growth factors. When you started to try to go over this normal restriction of proliferation the cells become like tumor cells. They express oncogenes and we don't know what they are becoming to do, and so we can be very cautious about the stimulation of endothelial cells proliferation, we can go over what is our goal and so it's something we have to look at.

Hanson: There is another strategy for promoting the healing of vascular grafts, and that is to enhance the formation of capillaries across the graft wall in order to seed the flow surface with endothelium. With more porous Teflon grafts this strategy has worked very nicely in primates. A similar study has been attempted in man which unfortunately gave negative results for reasons that we don't yet understand.

Mulvihill: Possibly for the same reasons that endothelial cells will not grow in a stenosis, they would not be capable of growing through capillaries either.

Hanson: Perhaps. However, if we could identify the appropriate growth factors which promote angiogenesis, and put them in the graft, we might stimulate such a process. This has not yet been tried.

Kieffer: Vascular smooth muscle cells might also be of great importance. There are close interactions between endothelial cells and smooth muscle cells. Especially the cytokine-mediated cellular crosstalk between both cell types might be necessary for a healthy and functional endothelium.

Wautier: It's a good question. I have not the answer. There is crosstalk between the cells. The most we know is between endothelial cells and smooth muscle cells but obviously there is some reverse influence. The matrix or the subendothelium is partly dependent from the products which are synthetized by some cells but also which come from smooth muscle cells and which induce differentiation. The cerebral vessels which have tight junction are very different from the other vessels. If in culture you use neural cells or you co-culture neural cells and endothelial cells coming from the aorta you reproduce the junction. So, there is obviously some influence between the non endothelial cells and the endothelial cells.

Davies: Do we think enough about how grafts are put in? Yannis, you raised this issue ten or fifteen minutes ago. Perhaps we think too much about the nature of the surfaces that we are implanting?

For the most part vascular grafts and heart valves function extremely well, even though the surfaces attract fibrinogen and platelets. They continue to function if the internal diameter of the lumen is large enough. Perhaps many of the failures that we have with bigger grafts and the failures that occur more frequently with small diameter grafts arise because of problems where the graft joins the normal vessel. We know if we're setting up systems, circuits or whatever to study these problems, that all the difficulties arise at the points where you join the bits and pieces together. That's where you generate shear stresses, and so stitches, differences in diameter between graft and vessel and the fact that the graft, unlike the vessel, is not pulsatile, is going to give rise to a lot of problems at the point where the graft and the normal vessel join. Maybe a lot of the residual difficulty with intravascular prostheses tends to arise at the points of insertion. What's happening in the middle of the graft is to a greater or a lesser extent irrelevant.

Missirlis: In a recent article in the Journal of Biomechanics by Lyman it was suggested that the impedance properties of the graft should match as closely as possible those of the vessel that it is attached. Otherwise even a very small difference would create down stream conditions that would generate some types of secondary flows that would initiate phenomena that you wish to avoid. And most studies have been done on cylindrical tubes while, for example, coronaries are tapered, so tapering is also a fact that should be taken into account. And the impedance matching really failled in the area where they were sutured. And this is something that I've heard surgeons talking in meetings that it is a very important paremeter: how you suture.

Therefore a fluid mechanical problem or a combination of such problems most probably is a starting point for events. Do you think so?

12. Hemorheological parameters

Hanson: I agree with this, and also think that the materials problem may be overestimated in some cases. We have taken conventional clinical grafts and have coated them by radiofrequency discharge methods with ultrathin layers of various polymers so as only change their surface chemical properties and not their texture, porosity, or handling characteristics. After implantation in animals for three months we evaluated these grafts for the development of anastomotic lesions and intimal thickening due to smooth muscle cell proliferation. We found no differences whatsoever between the different modified and control grafts, arguing that material surface properties may be in fact less important than other factors such as compliance mismatch.

Mulvihill: Just a point in support of this observation. We found when we inserted shunts into rats, in which the vascular system is much finer than in humans, we needed a very good surgeon to do the suture points correctly. When our student started this work, initially he found that using a silicone shunt these grafts would be patent for about 2 hr, but with a little practice two or three months later he could obtain grafts patent for 10 or 12 hr. It was simply a question of technique and good suturing to create a joint as smooth as possible. He also achieved better reproducibility in the patency, so experience is most important. The problem arises firstly at the joints. This can also be demonstrated by inserting a graft shunt in an animal and then radiolabelling platelets, fibrinogen or other blood components. A peak in platelet deposition or fibrinogen adsorption generally occurs at the anastomoses, particularly at the inlet end rather than the outlet end, as shows up if you analyse segment by segment when you explant the graft.

Missirlis: Could the question of how to improve biomaterials with respect to platelet interactions become more specific? How can one measure the biomaterial properties with respect to platelet interaction? Does it refer to platelets or to biomaterials? What I am trying to say: are we going to get a surface, and then platelets, and try to see how they interact? Am I making myself clear? Proteins are involved, platelets are involved, fluid mechanics are involved, mechanical properties are involved, how are we going to put this together with respect to platelet interactions? And I am asking the clinical people: what they would like to see and say: Well this is good for my platelets?

Y. F. Missirlis and J.-L. Wautier (eds.), The Role of Platelets in Blood-Biomaterial Interactions, 153–165.

Wautier: I think we come back to the point I raised before the better surface is the endothelial cell but it's not only a problem of surface it's also some secreted products which limited platelet interaction. You should have a surface which is the better we can have and also you have to have some products which limit platelet function in that part of the artificial circulation. I think we need both things. And so we need not only that the surface is good by itself or the better but can be but also that you have to minimise the accumulation of platelet.

Missirlis: When I receive some new polymeric tubes to test, and meanwhile we make up platelet rich plasma or a platelet solution, how much have we already interfered with these platelets?

Wautier: Well, I think that the first mistake is that we have worked for years with isolated platelets, washed plateletes, very neat platelets and that never happens *in vivo* so I think a system like the one described by Steve Hanson is a good system, you should have all the blood componenets there. It's how it is *in vivo*. And if you have only well washed platelets in buffer and look how they stick to something it never happens.

Davies: But the problem is one of practicality, isn't it? Probably the baboon model is one of the best that anybody has come up with for looking at artificial surfaces. But it's not a cheap and easy option. And if we are going to start from scratch by looking at all new biomaterials in the baboon shunt model it's going to be totally impractical. We have to work backwards. I agree that the best way to look at the performance of an intravascular graft is to implant it in an animal as close as possible to man and eventually implant it in man. With the most promising materials you would try experiments in which you grafted them into animals, looked at their characteristics and how long they remain patent for. Working backwords you end up looking for the same characteristics which determine long term patency using some kind of circuit, pumping blood, or modified blood, through a tube or the material that you are interested in. I don't see how you get away from that as being the fisrt step. Now one difficulty which we would all acknowledge is that the ideal fluid to be putting through these grafts is whole blood, but if you're going to do it with whole blood, you have to anticoagulate it in some way. Whether you have anticoagulated whole blood or blood components which have been artificially separated the artifact seems to me to be similar.

Wautier: I agree but there is a very simple system which has been deviced by all the people. That just when you collect blood just put the needle and you can have all the artificial material without any anticoagulant. And after that you can collect the blood in a tube and anticoagulate this blood to do the test you want. But you can have a look at a very short length of biomaterial and compare one to the other. It is not a model in an animal or in primates but it could be a cheaper, easier approach to test some of the materials in absence of anticoagulant and with whole blood.

Lemm: Duddley developed such a test, which is simply a bleeding test. A needle is inserted in the ear vein of a rabbit, a small diameter tube is connected and the time is measured until bleeding has stopped.

Hanson: These tests might be suitable for first level screening. For example, tubes that occlude very quickly might be excluded from further consideration on this basis. My concern about many *in vitro* tests is that they are highly unlikely to predict later events that could be very important, for example, the involvement of white cells. However, *in vitro* testing could be useful for screening materials intended for short term applications, such as certain catheters.

Davies: From your experience, do you have a feel for what the ideal preliminary screening tests are? You probably have more experience than any of us in looking at whole animal methods of evaluating biomaterials so you must have some thoughts about the best methods to study blood-biomaterials interaction at an earlier stage in the process of evaluation.

Hanson: This has been very frustrating. First, you need to consider the device application and perhaps the best test is to evaluate devices in their intended usage configuration. One needs to simulate local blood flow conditions, and duration of blood exposure. There are also questions about the relevance of different animal models. No test addresses all these issues satisfactorily. We would not claim that our primate studies necessarily predict clinical outcomes, although we are trying to establish such correlations. So, at this point I cannot recommend any *in vitro* or *ex vivo* tests that would be predictive, because we don't know that they are.

Davies: That's the sad fact isn't it? Forty years experience of working collectively in this field and we still really do not have the correlation betweeen the simple, initial screening test and what happens even in animal models, let alone what happens in man.

Wautier: The strategy which has been used for drugs : the first screening : is the drug active? Second : is it toxic in animals or in cell culture? Third : one trial in human and second, third stages is have not been conducted in the same way for biomaterials. I think it's probably the way to do it? To have the same steps. First is this material very toxic? Is it interesting or not? Second in a long term animal study it works. Starting from cheap animals and go further in primates and at the end men. I think we have to follow the same strategy. Otherwise we could be, if we are still alive, in twenty years from now and have the same absence of correlation between *in vitro* tests and *in* *vivo* situation.

Mulvihill: Concerning the *ex vivo* test as a preliminary screening test, I think this has possibilities. However, with regard to experimental technique, we found that you have to be very careful about flow conditions. These can vary: if you simply implant a catheter into a number of individuals, you will find a very different flow rate according to the vascular tree of the person. I myself, for instance, am a hopeless subject for a catheter because I have a slow blood flow rate and it blocks up very quickly, whereas other subjects can give much better results. Likewise, if you follow the generation of FPA in non anticoagulated blood flowing from such a catheter, the delay time to the moment at which major FPA generation starts and the blood begins to clot varys according to the individual. In one volunteer the delay may be 3 min, in another 8 min. The result is highly reproducible if you do the same test on the same person but it will vary from person to person. So you require quite a number of volunteers for this kind of test. We try in our *ex vivo* system to avoid the anticoagulant problem by minimising anticoagulant levels and we place a pump at some point in the circuit so as to give a constant flow rate, which with a constant diameter of the catheter enables some standardisation of the screening test. Otherwise we have found very poor results even as a preliminary test.

Wautier: This system is done every day on thousands of people, when they are blood donors for apheresis. There is line, there is pump and so it's done everday on thousands of people and it has never been used just to evaluate if the tubing which is used in this situation is good and we know exactly what are the parameters of what is the blood flow and all these things can be calculated very easily and this has never been conducted in a large scale.

Lemm: Biomaterials are used in two different ways: for longterm and short-term applications. For economical reasons difficult chemical procedures in order to modify the surfaces of disposal materials must be excluded. Yesterday you mentioned in connection with blood bags an improved PVC with a new type of plasticiser as well as a new polyolefine. Are these alternative materials significantly more expensive than traditional materials?

Wautier: I think the cost is between 2.5 and 3 times higher than the P.V.C. products? It is one of the limitations. I don't know why it is so expensive, for technical reasons or the limitation of the market.

Lemm: In fact, the reason is the price. But PVC is so cheap because it is used in enormous quantities. In terms of hemocompatibility PVC is a rather good material but polyurethanes are better. However, their price is a hundred times higher than the price for PVC. Therefore, health insurances will not cover the costs for blood bags or tubings made of polyurethanes.

Wautier: Could we expect later. If I remember well teflon was discovered and now we have teflon everywhere, we have in cooking system, and it surprises us probably it increased tremendously in five, ten years time. Could we expect that for other materials that the same thing will happen? If the material will be used in a more large scale for other purpose that only biomaterial interest of the product.

Lemm: In general big chemical companies are not interested in the production of medical polymers because the quantities to be produced are too small. Other companies do not want to assume the responsibility and the risk for the production of medical grade materials.

Wautier: I don't know anything about how to build cars but I saw TV and they were telling they were producing new cars with new, more deformable materials. So what is going on in the other fields were the market is bigger and they are using more and more synthethic products. I don't know if the products they are making could have some interest or could have some side products for us.

Lemm: Economical reasons are an argument against the production of better hemocompatible materials.

Mulvihill: Certainly economics always enter into the question. For instance, in some dialysis clinics the patients are screened. It is now known that the original dialysers based on cuprophan membranes tend to activate the complement system. Hence for older patients the clinics will use cuprophan dialysers, whereas for younger ones they will prefer polysulphone. The cost is higher but for a younger subject they consider this to be worthwhile and unfortunately the choice is made on an age and economic basis. This is nevertheless the reality of the situation.

Davies: We have to accept that life is based on economics. We could do more for the health of the world and all go home tomorrow just by raising the income of people in developing countries. Even if you are thinking of the greatest good of the greatest number, you still have to consider the economics of cardiovascular implants. I was very interested in the point you made, which has never struck me, that from the point of view of the chemical polymer companies the medical market is so small that they would not make or develop materials specifically for that end unless thay were of a very high added value.It seems to me that the implication of what you were saying is that we are speculating in a vacuum, because even if we do decide there are better kinds of materials that we might use for these purposes, unless they happen also to be good for making synthetic clothes or plastic car bodies we are not going to get them because the companies won't make them.

Missirlis: I am not so sure.

Lemm: This is what we observe in Germany. The big companies are not interested in these fields.

Missirlis: Yes, but maybe a small company could do it because in contrary to your angument I heard the other day that Dow Chemical Company in the U.S.A. desided not to market anymore the silicon prosthesis because of "problems", and I heard that 1% of its income comes only from this prosthesis. So economics is a "must" but people make heart valves, which is a small market in terms of material production but the cost is high so if there is a market you can produce whatever you wish and the cost will go higher, and people would pay for it.

Davies: Yes, we know that. But there is a difference between a high value added product like a heart valve and everyday objects like blood bags and giving sets. The harsh economics of health care delivery, even in the richest countries, are going to dictate that because PVC is cheap and available, we use it. If big companies are not prepared to produce better compounds in bulk, small companies are going to be charging a huge amount extra for a marginally better product.

You can justify the additional cost when it is a high value added product. But for an everyday, cheap product it's difficult to do that.

Missirlis: P.V.C. is also 50% chloride and if you dispose of this we don't know what whould happen after 50 years with so much chloride being dumped or burnt or whatever. So there are arguments even to change into non-chlorinated polymers in the medical and other markets, I think.

Wautier: That means that possible pollution by the use of chloride may limit the use of chloride, so that it could be a good argument to push in this direction.

Lemm: Dow Chemical decided to stop the production of the best hemocompatible polymer, the polyurethane "Pellethane", because it is a 100 times more expensive than the cheaper PVC and this is why there is no longer a market for Pellethane.

Wautier: Yes, but these things can change. I was in a discussion about recombinant products. About growth factors for the bone marrow which become now largely used. And when we discussed about 5 years ago with the big pharmaceutical companies they said : well, it's interesting but we will never market that. It's so expensive compared to the chemicals. Now there is a big market for this type of products. So these things can change in 4–5 years time. It is difficult to predict.

Hanson: I think that you first have to show that the new growth factor or the new polymer is clearly better. If you can show that, then I think the market may develop.

Mulvihill: This tends towards the situation where if there is a high added value to your product, as in the case of a heart valve, it is perhaps worth it for small scale production. If the product is clearly better, it is worth it. Possibly not for larger companies and it will perhaps always be difficult to convince the large chemical companies to produce this kind of device. You have to look to smaller companies who are limited to the medical domain. Then stimulate sufficient interest when you have a good product to convince them to market it.

Davies: But I think it is important that we keep these things in proportion. Dr. Hanson comes from a state close to the state which has attracted interest from around the world by starting to draw up a list of operations, diseases and procedures for which the state insurance will reimburse the doctors and hospitals. When the budget has been spent a line is drawn and other conditions which are of less cost-effectiveness are not covered.

The same thing is starting to happen in the UK and after all, we are talking about some of the wealthiest countries in the world. We are moving in the situation, in the UK, where the national health insurance is ceasing to cover minor operations. Now if into that mix we try to float the idea that we should interest more companies in making giving sets and blood collection bags that are three times more expensive than the ones we have already, we will have a problem of conviction.

Wautier: Yes, I think it is a crucial problem but I am not sure that all the things are managed on the political point. I understand that they don't be involved in the market of health, and that the market of health will self limited as all the markets. But I've a figure which stresses me is the amount of money that the French people use in a year for their car and for their health and it's similar: 9000F for their car and 9000F for their health. So could anybody tell you have to reduce the price of the car and not to have a car or two cars? I think that's a society. Would you prefer to be in a good health or to have two cars?

Lemm: I think we are to some extent dependent on industry, but on the other side we should not minimize our influence on the producers. I would like to remind you of the discussion on the two plasticisers in PVC. The new THETM (tri-(ethyl–2hexyl)-trimellitat) is a little more expensive than the traditional one DEHP (di-(ethyl–2hexyl)-phthalate), it is though more or less generally used. The cheap PVC basically needs plasticisers and other ingredients. Research should be done on the development of additives which are more biofriendly, which are able to interfere in a positive way with the coagulation system of blood. Such additives must be stable enough to survive the extrusion process. It is known that plasticisers which are chemically terminated with aspirin are able to tolerate temperature up to 200°C. Even with regard to economical considerations such an ingredient could be accepted.

I would like to repeat my question, what are the disadvantages you are facing daily in using blood bags, when you collect blood? What would you like to have improved?

Wautier: I think the first thing we will improve platelet storage is to have platelets that are kept in condition in which they will be active? I think this is the most important thing and few criteria could be recommended.

First is the condition, gas exchange, that's very traditionnal because it influences pH which appears to be crucial for keeping platelets in good condition. The other things which are not being well studied is the geometry or design of the bag appropriate for keeping the platelets in good condition. We agitate, and know that is better but is it the better size, the better shape of bags for keeping platelets? I think it's probably the more convenient for them just to seal a film of plastic material but could we have some ideas of how it could be better? Could we have better preservative for keeping the platelets in better condition during storage for short, or longer period of time? I think one of the limitations we have, when we keep platelets at 22 degrees, which apparently at the present time is the best temperature is the ageing if we can reduce the temperature we probably can minimize the rate of ageing. Could we have special containers which will be efficient with the appropriate preservative to keep platelets for a longer period of time than what we have now? What is done on this field is very poor and very little platelets which are frozen are efficient after the storage.

Lemm: But, are you dependent on using disposable materials?

Wautier: Yes.

Mulvihill: Has anyone ever tried reusing platelet storage bags?

Wautier: As I remember at the beginning blood was collected into glass containers and the first technique which was used to be able to separate platelets from the whole blood was siliconized glass but the centrifugation was a problem bad. The other problem was after that to separate the platelets in sterile conditions from a bottle of glass which was not achieved at that time. A closed system, sterile from the venipuncture to the last bag, in which platelets have to be collected has been a great improvement for the technology of platelet collection from one standard donation. For the cell separator I think the systems which are used now can be improved in terms of non-activating the platelets before collecting them apparently that has been told by some of us. It is present in the litterature that the tubing and all the collectors activate a part of the platelets which are collected and also leucocytes. And this is a disadvantage for having the platelets still ready for transfusion and efficient for the hemostatic system. So if we can have the line between the patient the donor with all the plasma collecting system and back to the donor with a surface which is non-activating surface for platelets it will be probably a great advantage. And I think that is the same problem for the other application we discuss about biomaterials, that the biomaterial has to be a non-activating surface for platelets, for graft, for extra-corporeal circulation. So the purpose is completely different but the goal is quite similar to have surface which have little activating properties for platelets.

Missirlis: Are the mechanical properties of platelet of importance to you. In other words: if you keep platelets say for 5 days in a bag, apart from their functional biological activity do you think that their integrity, their stability in terms of structure may be compromized? Would it be of interest to you to measure the mechanical properties of platelets? Do you think that is relevant from a clinical point of view?

Wautier: Yes. I think it is because we know that the mechanical properties as they are dependent upon the cyto-skeleton. A. Ordinas showed us yesterday some pictures. The capacity of platelets to change shape is also dependent upon the different intracellular metabolism, so the result of the mechanical properties could be dependent upon several parameters which are important for platelet function.

We are in the Pythagore island and I heard very little about the geometry of the tubing of the bags or all this things. We are not very creative in that field. We are making tubes which are very rigid, which do not correspond to our vessel, which we know, that they can change size, they can be irregular, they can have some differences in terms of geometry and also for the bags we're making the most simple product we can. They have plastic film they fold the film and seal it is that very appropriate. Could we have an annular geometry for the cells or for the blood. And possibly we can think about other geometrical form for the containers, for the tubings, that could be not that regular as we make two lines just straight, and which could improve the rheological parameters you described earlier. There could be a little difference. We know that "la loi de Poiseuille" is not true in the body, it is true in a tube but it's not true in the body. Could we change some of the aspects of the geometry which could make a difference in cell-cell interaction and in cell-biomaterial interactions?

Hanson: This is a good question, and I think one obvious variable might be the surface-to-volume ratio. If we think a surface is doing bad things, we can minimize it. In this context, a tube configuration would be much better that a flat bag. So I agree that device geometry could be very important in many instances.

Mulvihill: You must also consider the problem of gas exchange. If you change the surface to volume ratio you also modify the gas exchange properties, so it would be a question of the right balance between the two factors. With regard to tubing inlet and outlet, I think the best configuration would be the simplest possible in order to avoid problems of turbulence, because it's always when you have a complicated configuration that you strike difficulties in these flow systems. Perhaps a straight tube is not too bad after all.

Wautier: Could we imagine other forms in which the surface construction could be different. They are changing shape to adapt their volume towards what they have to go through. I think that the nature is very economic and when the nature has found a system which is working it tries to keep the system. And when we are looking at what is happening in our vessel which we know to be best it is not a very simple geometry.

In addition there are a lot of I can not say drugs, but mediators to minimize the interaction. In terms of material we can improve to a certain extent, but I know very little research which has been conducted to try to have different shapes for the containers, for the tubing and this type of things.

Missirlis: I have never thought about it in this way. When you have a bag full of cells in their solution medium, I thought that one should keep the metabolism as low as possible so that you have the minimum of reactions, and it is a matter of space and handling (because nurses are going to take it from here to there). So the problems of hemodynamics I considered mostly in designing the artificial organs, or grafts, or valves, where actually for long times (even for catheters etc.) you are going to have interaction of flowing blood within or around such a structure. But in storage I am sure that the platelets that sit on the surface would react differently than those in the centre. Now, whether you need to have them agitated inside, whether you need to have as few contacting the surface as possible, whether during the collection you must have as laminar a flow as possible, so that you don't shear them enough to generate release products that would start activating in the bag, these are, I think, mostly collection problems, that is how a nurse collects, rather than design a tube more similar to the natural case. Because, there, the mechanics of the cardiovascular system are not just to minimize the shear stress but to propagate the pulse wave and the fluid with the minimum energy from the heart out through the circulatory system. So the way that the arterial system is constructed is not just to interact with the blood elements in the least disturbing way but also to mechanically propagate blood down the system. But in terms of collection bags I don't know what happens to the many billions of cells you have there. While they are sitting at 4–20°C should they be agitated all the time?

Wautier: It has been observed that they are better preserved, when they are agitated rather than when they are not. I don't know the exact explanation. It's proposed, that during agitation there is a better gas exchange but I'm not sure this is the only explanation. In a country we are making wine. We know that wine is not kept in the same conditions, according to the size of the bottle, to the way you put the bottle horizontal or vertical makes a huge difference because of gas exchange, and also the colour of the container, the size of the container could play some role I don't know what is the effect on the light on the platelet preservation. Is it better to put them in the dark or not? There are many many things which have never, been properly studied and which can possibly not be, the way we are speaking about cost, but that, possibly, can not increase the cost tremendously and can improve the things easily.

Kieffer: You just mentioned that platelets used for transfusion can be stored from 4 to 20°C. However, it is known that low temperature activates platelets. I wonder whether there is a difference in the survival time of transfused platelets that have been stored at 4 or 20°C.

Wautier: In our hands, we have studied platelets stored at 4 degrees and 20 degrees the last appears to be better. Actually there are several reports, which are difficult to argue against, that assure that if you store platelets at 4 degrees and you look at the *in-vitro* function of these cells they have been altered but if you inject these platelets and look at the platelets survival they have better platelets survival than the platelets that have been stored at 20 degrees. It appears on several tests that 20°C is better than 4 degrees but there is not a general agreement on that. It's 2/3 of the workers who say it's better at 20 degrees and 1/3 that's better at 4 degrees. It's not scientifically completely established.

Kieffer: The long tubing on the platelet transfusion bags is certainly also an important factor responsible for platelet activation. For the purpose of good quality platelets, it would be better to have platelet transfusion bags with shorter tubings.

Davies: Well, it's practical because patients like to move their arms around and an even worse thing for the clinician is to find the patient has pulled the drip down by moving their arms. So you need to have a long tube unless you stick the bag to the patient and then it starts to get comlicated.

Missirlis: But is the surface area-to-volune ratio argument against the agitation, I mean...

Wautier: No, it's not against it.

Hanson: It just means that you have more surface area of polymer for platelets to interact with. Questions of bag agitation, surface area, and flow phenomena may be balanced by requirements for gas exchange and other factors.

Davies: The theory of your argument is incontrovertible but if the surface is bad the less surface you have, the better. And so clearly on theoretical grounds the closer the bag gets to a perfect sphere the better your surface-volume relationship will be. This needs to be referred back to our colleagues on the biomaterials side but I would quess that the cost of making a cylindrical or circular bag would actually be considerably higher, because of the way you seal the two films of plastic together if it is a sphere or a cylinder. You've got to have much more complicated joints at the end of a cylinder or around a sphere and you've also got to have your inlet for the needle. So I would guess that it would be quite an expensive option, but I don't want to replay the economics angument.

Hanson: If you take a conventional bag and fill it, it can become nearly cylindrical or spherical. So, by near complete filling of perhaps smaller bags made in the conventional way you might achieve the same thing.

Missirlis: I still haven't understood when you agitate don't you create fluid forces that would bring a platelet more into contact with the surface rather than non-agitation? What do you mean by agitation?

Ordinas: To store bag platelets it has been proven that continuous agitation is required and in the past several apparatus were designed to this purpose. Some had circular movements while others made side-to-side movements and in others the movement was that of rotation.

Davies: But we don't really know what it's doing, it's just empirical.

Wautier: That's not been demonstrated in keeping the platelets in.

Ordinas: At this point in the discussion I think it would be interesting to explain exactly what the procedure is to obtain a platelet bag. You start with a whole blood bag from a single donor with three satellite bags which are connected by tube to the first bag. The four bags are centrifuged and red blood cells remain in the first bag and platelet rich plasma (PRP) is then passed into the first of the three satellite bags which are then disconnected from the first bag. The three satellite bags are centrifuged again and from the PRP the platelet concentrate is obtained and the supernatant, platelet poor plasma (PPP) is passed into the second satellite bag and disconnected. At this point the remaining two satellite bags may undergo one of two options: freeze the PPP or continue the procedure to obtain cryoprecipitate.

The platelet concentrate from the first satellite bag is left in a resting state due to the aggregation of the platelets produced by the centrifugation. The platelets rest for one hour to obtain complete disaggregation. At this point the platelets are put under agitation.This is the procedure used in our Hospital.

Missirlis: Are all these bags sterilised by ethylenoxide?

Wautier: I think yes.

Missirlis: Has somebody studied the effect of the sterilisation agent on the viability of platelets?

Wautier: No, we know that there is some chemical reaction on some leakage from the plasticiser but to what extent it is affecting the cell viability or the cell function has not been studied.

Missirlis: Do you worry about it?

Wautier: I think we have to worry but the people are worrying more if the volume of this product which is infused in the patients who receive iterative transfusion. But know that to a certain level it's toxic for liver.

Ordinas: At present it would be of great interest to produce new plastic materials for the designing of new bags which would provide greater benefits. I realize that from an economical point of view this would represent a large market if a less expensive bag, but with the same advantages, could be produced. Recently, our Hospital tried out a new, less expensive bag, with blood donors. However, it seems that the manufacturer had not taken the needle into account and in the end the donor complained because of the bad needle and the previously used, more expensive bags, had to be used.

13. Modulation of platelet functions

Davies: I wonder whether anybody here knows anything about what it is that happens to platelets when you rest them. I remember a little from the work of Joachim Reimers working in Fraser Mustard's laboratory on the properties of thrombin-degranulated platelets. These platelets, during thrombin treatment, had a pretty rough time and one of the phases in resuscitating them, as with the platelets in blood bags, was just to leave them to sit on the bench for twenty minutes. Maybe that is also the explanation why platelets which, if you characterise them in the bag, don't seem to be terribly good, and when you transfuse them back into the patient work better again. This ability that platelets have to be able to restore their physiological function after a difficult experience in a bag or elsewhere, is something that enables us to get away with things in storage for platelet transfusion which otherwise wouldn't erable us to do it. But I dont't think anybody knows very much about what's happening to the platelet.

Wautier: Do you mean for desaggregation?

Davies: No, I mean what is happening in this time when you leave the bag on the bench. Why, when Joachim Reimers was making his thrombin-degranulated platelets did he leave them for 20 min?

You leave slightly damaged platelets to sit for a little, and they function very much better. Well, I wonder what's happening?

Wautier: I don't have the exact explanation but there was a study which has been made using CP/CPK additive which shows that we can reverse the effect of ADP on platelets agreggation and after addition of CP/CPK they can be reaggregated by a next addition of ADP. We know that the shape of the plaletet is something which can be reversibly modified and if there is not a strong link between two platelets this can be reversible. When you leave platelets after the stress they have been exposed during the centrifugation they can recover their normal shape.

Mulvihill: Did you say that these platelets not only recovered their functional capacity but also their granules? This amazes me because I have always understood that once a platelet was degranulated it was degranulated for the rest of its life. Being a non nucleated cell, it will not be able to resynthesize the products which have been lost. Was there any evidence produced microscopically or in other ways to show that granules were reformed?

Y. F. Missirlis and J.-L. Wautier (eds.), The Role of Platelets in Blood-Biomaterial Interactions, 167–180.

Wautier: This work is quite old, it's from the 70's and it was really unexpected that the platelets can recover granule after they have been degranulated. But we cannot extrapolate from rabbits, to human. We know that rabbit platelets the granules contain a high amount of histamin while there is very little histamin in human platelets. So, possibly the physiology of platelets in rabbits is a little different from the human.

Mulvihill: Has anybody tried putting apyrase in conservation bags? We know that platelets in suspension tend to generate low levels of ADP and one method of improving storage of washed platelets is to put apyrase into the medium to degrade this ADP.

Wautier: I think apyrase was used *in vitro* but you know apyrase is not that easy to purify? Even if you have a ton of potatoes it's not that easy to produce pure apyrase. And I'm not sure it's innocent to infuse apyrase in human, so that has been just tested *in vitro*. And the reasons why investigators look at CP/CPK it's that it was going along the same line and they prefer to use CP/CPK since it appears not to be as toxic as apyrase.

Lemm: I would like to discuss another point: surface modifications of blood bags, tubings and other disposable materials. Yesterday, you mentioned specific drugs protecting platelets. What kind of specific receptors for pharmaceutical drug would you like to have on the surface of a new material? I imagine a simple procedure: you inject a pharmaceutical drug just before you use the blood bag or similar devices and the drug binds to the surface pre-activated with a specific receptor. The efficiency of such a surface modification must not exceed five days.

Hanson: Which type of device do you specifically refer to?

Lemm: I refer to tubings and storage bags.

Wautier: You showed that probably thrombin generation is important. Do you think that it will be important to try to minimize thrombin generation during storage?

Davies: How much evidence is there that we have got thrombin activation. What's the background FPA (fibrinopeptide A) concentration or TAT (thrombin-antithrombin) complex concentration in a bag with whole blood after 48 hr or 72 hr. We suspect that acid citrate dextrate would be failry effective in suppressing it.

Wautier: We are not sure of that. Because you must be sure that ACD is going everywhere and we don't have any leukocyte which is starting to produce tissue factor somewhere.

Davies: I accept that the knowledge may be available somewhere but it isn't available to us at this moment. But citrate is a fairly effective anticoagulant at a high concentration because so much coagulation is calcium-dependant.

Wautier: That is right.

Davies: If we are concentrating on platelets, then I would have thought that the process is feasible and achievable. PGI_2 would have to be the front runner because we know it's a very effective platelet inhibitor, and it inhibits both adhesion and aggregation. We know that the effect will go with time, so that the platelets would be effective when you transfuse them. Obviously if you have an inhibitor that is permanent and knocks out all the platelets that may keep them looking nice in the bag but they are not much use when you give them to the patient. And we know that PGI_2 is safe when administered to human beings at the doses that inhibit platelet function. And as I understand it, it's already technically achievable to put PGI_2 onto certain polymer surfaces. So I would have thought that for a number of reasons PGI_2 would be the most attractive compound to put onto polymers for blood storage and certainly for platelet transfusion bags.

Hanson: I don't think that we know what the real problem in blood storage is. If it's thrombin generation, it may not be related to the surface and you could add soluble hirudin or some other antithrombin to block that specific mechanism. If it's related to the surface, then we might want to block cell adhesion and I'm not sure how we would do that.

Mulvihill: Has anybody tried to immobilize protein C or activated protein C on a surface?

Hanson: I'm not aware of studies with immobilized protein C. One could also consider immobilizing thrombomodulin.

Lemm: And what do you think about immobilized aspirin?

Davies: I would not see aspirin is a good canditate because you are going permanently to inhibit some of the functions of platelets. It's not a reversible effect.

Lemm: Aspirin is known to be a specific receptor for albumin, it binds albumin.

Davies: I see, you are thinking of it as a way to linking albumin. I thought you were thinking of it as a way to preserve platelet function. I know nothing about its effect on binding albumin. I have to say that I don't think from the clinical point of view – maybe Jean-Luc would disagree with me – and

I accept that there is an increasing requirement for platelet transfusion but, I don't think that this a big problem in clinical practice. I think one of the difficulties that suppliers of blood products face, as with all clinical laboratory sercices, is that if you offer clinicians a service they overuse it, so I suspect that most patients who require platelet transfusions are given more platelets than are required. And I doubt whether there is a really big problem that we should be trying to solve in transfusion of platelets which are not very active.

Wautier: There could be some arguments to support the idea that the prescription of platelets could be a little higher than what it's striktly required? One of the main reasons for that is that we cannot guarantee the quality of the product which is transfused. If we can tell a clinician you can transfuse 5 units of platelets and you will have no risk of a hemorragic problem they will do that. But at the present time with the difficulty we have to assess a real efficiency of platelet collected in different conditions stored for different times, they prescribe twice the amount usually recommended for a patient. So, I think if the quality of platelets will be more standardized the number of units of platelets which will be transfused will be reduced.

Davies: I'm unconvinced about that. I think the problem is that you're dealing with two kinds of human recipient. The sort of recipient in whom you are going to carry out the studies (I mean if you are going to do platelet survival or bleeding times, or whatever it is – and we are going to talk about that later), is going to be more-or-less in a stable condition, or you are going to choose patients who are not bleeding but are thrombocytopenic.

The problem comes in people who are bleeding, or in treating patients with leukaemia and thrombocytopenia who need massive platelet tranfusions. Their bleeding problem is usually catastrophic and not easy to characterise. So clinicians give many units of platelets to these patients because they want to put the problem right. They don't have to measure when enough is enough, so they give too much. And I suspect that a lot of platelet transfusion is actually given on an empirical basis, because we don't know what intermediate measurements of platelet function to accept and that would enable us to give the right amount and no more. If you are giving fresh frozen plasma, for example, to someone who had an overdose of warfarin, you can keep measuring the prothrombin time. But giving platelets to people, you cannot say to the clinician, give enough platelets to achieve ..... to achieve what? Some level of platelet count? We talked about this yesterday. Yes we can specify a certain platelet count, but maybe the platelets you're counting are not so great functionally.

Mulvihill: I think if they are not function they can be possibly eliminated.

Wautier: You are a bit pessimistic. There is a consensus about when platelets have to be transfused and there are different criteria. In brief the criteria are platelet count, hemorrhagic problems, infection, chemotherapy, a major surgery or minor intervention. All these things have to be taken into account and you decide what are the indications of platelet transfusion. I think it is quite clear. I'm not sure that all the clinicians respect these rules. To evaluate what is the efficacy of the platelet transfusion in a patient the easiest way and the cheapest way beside the clinical observation of the arrest of bleeding, is to measure platelet count one hour after transfusion. You can calculate what is the increment in the platelet count. That is not a gold standard but it's a good indicator of how the platelets recirculate and if you can expect some efficacy of the platelet transfusion. So I will not be so pessimistic about that. But what is true is that when there was no platelet transfusion or very little platelet transfusion most of the patient with leukemia died from cerebral hemorrage. Now it's rare. There was a big progress made in that area. But now for a clinician who is in charge of a patient with leukemia he cannot accept that the patient dies from hemorrhage. So there is a tendency that on Saturday they prescribe a heavy transfusion not to be nervous during the weekend. That's true but it's something which is difficult to avoid, I guess.

Davies: I think we actually agree with each other. If you can say to a clinician to give enough platelets to achieve a circulating count of 50×10^9 or whatever, and that was generally acceptable, then you could make that the goal of platelet transfusion therapy. And then we could go back and look at the problem of the bags and the shape of the bags and everything else and say: Look at the relative volume you need to achieve, to have 50000 circulating platelets per microlitre one hour later. But we don't generally accept that, I suspect because the data that relate platelet number to cessation of clinical bleeding are not as strong as all that. I certainly accept what you say, that the availability of platelet transfusion has transformed the treatment and improved the survival of bleeding patients who are severely thrombocytopenic. There is no doubt about that at all. But this comes back to the point where I started, with which Dr. Ordinas agrees, that in clinical practice there is not a big residual problem. Adequate platelet transfusion is very effective in stopping people dying from thrombocytopenia.

Wautier: There are too much units of platelets used. And that's a risk of alloimmunisation to transmit disease which is unacceptable to my point of view. If we know exactly the number of functional platelets we transfused we can minimise the number of units we transfuse. The benefit for the patient is obvious and from the economical point is also an economy because if you reduce the number of the units you reduce the cost of the treatment.

Davies: Can you tell us what the present percentage utilization of transfused platelets is? Do you have any kind of figure whether you get 30% still circulating at an hour or ...

Wautier: I would say that the situation at the present time is very disappointing because you don't know exactly what is the number of platelets in one bag. So that's the first thing which is for me very important. And besides there are some aggregates which will be stopped at the filter and never go to the patient. That's the second point. It's difficult to evaluate in the present condition what is the exact number of the platelets which are really infused to the patient. But I would say from the economical point of view in the Hôpitaux de Paris which consist in several hospitals and all the hospitals together is the biggest hospital in Europe, the first cost for transfusion is platelet transfusion. There was a big reduction in red blood cell transfusion and in plasma transfusion and now for surgery they are more and more using autotransfusion, but platelet transfusion are still increasing. So in terms of the economy of the Hospital it's not a point you can avoid.

Kieffer: Is it important in platelet transfusion to consider histocompatibility and platelet specific alloantigens, and is a crossmatch test with the patient's serum and the donor's platelets necessary?

Wautier: It is only considered when the patients have iterative platelet transfusions I mean when you transfuse platelets and there is no increment in platelet count. And it's only taken into account in this condition or if a patient should have bone marrow transplantation or platelet congenital disorders. Otherwise it's not taken into account. There is a study which was conducted in Canada where they evaluated the cost effectiveness of pretransfusion test before and the efficacy of the transfusion. They found that the association of two tests can predict the efficacy of transfusion of the patients who are immunised.

Hanson: We have performed studies in which donor platelets were labeled with Chromium–51 and transfused into patients with thrombocytopenia due to bone marrow hypoplasia. Most of those platelets circulated with near normal lifespan, although those platelets were usually just harvested and had not been stored for long periods.

Davies: We're talking about an incremental improvement of something around 75% You're assuming there is not a great loss in the bag of the most viable platelets. What you are saying is that all our discussion for the last couple of hours has been trying to achieve an incremental increase in the number of ...

Hanson: And trying to prolong the storage life. Fresh platelets work best, while longer storage periods cause platelet dysfunction. I would ask the question: Are we certain that there is a biomaterials problem with platelet storage?

Wautier: It's difficult to know what is the main factor. There is some activation of platelets during storage. Is it due to the biomaterial and the change of the biomaterial could improve that, that's a question I cannot answer myself. We know that switching from glass to plastic there was a huge difference. Could we move to a second or third generation of plastics that keep platelets better that's an open question.

Hanson: I think the plastic can make a difference. Certainly the early generation PVC bags contained plasticizers and leachable additives that were not very helpful. The question may be whether the present generation bags could be further improved.

Davies: I'm sure it's improved, but in all these things there is an asymptotic approach to perfection and I suspect we are already pretty high on the curve of acceptability of these bags. And I wonder whether putting a great deal of energy into improving what we have is worth it, but I don't know the answer.

Mulvihill: If adequate platelet transfusion is achieved with the present bags, possibly it is of greater interest to develop better biomaterials for other applications, where the quality of the material is more critical, for instance vascular implants and extracorporeal circulation systems where we have obvious problems. If these bags already function well and as you say could only possibly be improved at considerable cost, is it really worth it?

Wautier: I am sure it's more dramatic to have the occlusion of an artificial vessel than to have an accident with inefficiency of platelet transfusion, but when we count in terms of health policy the number of transfusions which are made compared to the implantation of artificial graft there is no comparison between. The difference is too big. What I've said is that we don't know exactly what is the importance of biomaterial, what is the respective effect of preservative/biomaterial/tubing. We are very happy we are doing our best, everything is nice but I'm not sure we cannot improve all these things and I'm not sure also that there will be a great increase in the cost because possibly by simple modification of the shape of the bag, the addition of a little of PGI_2 or a little citrate we can improve tremendously the efficacy of the platelets and can store them for more than 24 hr. We know platelets are good when used within 24 hr but when you have a long weekend or when you can't have blood donors at the right time you don't have enough platelets and we must try to expand the time we can keep platelets in a better condition.

Lemm: I would like to raise a final question: Do you have any experience with the elements of Rare Earth? In litterature they are mentioned to prevent blood coagulation, it is however, not known, where they actually interface the cascade. A pharmaceutical drug based on Neodym was available on the market but disappeared after a few years. Do you have any information whether these metals are toxic?

Wautier: The only thing I know is not a rear metal but it's Lithium. Lithium has been shown many years ago to modify platelet function. It's also used as a treatment but it's also toxic so you have to minimize the amount of Lithium that could be added. But as far as I remember the concentration of Lithium which has to be used to modify platelet function was quite limited.

Lemm: In fact, the efficiency of Neodym is not very high in comparison to Heparin or other coagulants but we picked up the idea to fix it on a surface. With such an immobilized metal on the surface we will not have nay sterilization problems; we might expose such materials to any procedure which is tolerated by the polymer itself.

Wautier: I think that would be very important for leucocyte adhesion which is very dependent upon ions and if you put some metals they can compete with normal ions like Calcium or Magnesium. For example if you put Manganese in the system it blocks the normal adhesion. So for leucocyte interaction that possibly could be a reason to search. For platelets the other thing I know is the story about Lithium.

Lemm: So, you do not know what kind of mechanism it could be.

Wautier: There is another possibility in molecular level in which this product could interfere with it the metabolism.

Ordinas: This will be the last session and I am pleased to chair this discussion because I am sure that what we are about to discuss is in the mind of all those present. The title of this session is " Limitation of measurements of platelet parameters". Eary this morning, Prof. Missirlis asked whether there was any good test to evaluate and predict the interaction of platelets with foreign surfaces and whether this surface would be more, or less reactive, as a result of this test,than other surfaces already in the market. I think that this is a good point to start the discussion and ask everybody present whether they agree that an *in vitro* test is able to predict what is expected *in vivo*.

Hanson: My opinion is that *in vitro* tests may not predict *in vivo* events, except for certain gross phenomena. For example, surfaces that potently activate intrinsic coagulation *in vitro* may not be suitable for some applications where rapid thrombosis is a problem. Such applications might include very small diameter blood conduits which could fail within minutes to hours. *in vitro* testing might predict these short-term outcomes, but probably cannot predict later events including fibrinolytic processes, the reactions of white cells, and thrombus reorganization. These mechanisms probably affect long-term patency of vascular grafts, the frequency of embolism from artificial heart valves, etc. So the *in vitro* tests may be perhaps be useful in the first-order screening of materials for certain short-term applications.

Materials should also be studied in their actual usage configuration whenever possible, with due regard for the blood flow conditions. So, there may not simply be good materials and bad materials. Results may depend on the surface configuration and flow environment. In our studies, textured surfaces invariably accumulate platelets and fibrin, while smooth surfaces of the same polymer may be quite nonreactive. When you avoid surface texture and roughness, even procoagulant surfaces like glass may be non-thrombogenic if the blood flow is rapid. Thus, since surface chemistry, texture, device geometry, and flow conditions are all important variables, we cannot classify materials as simply good or bad generally.

Lemm: In *in vitro* tests you can use human blood.

Ordinas: I think that these kinds of experiments must always be carried out with whole blood since, in the past, a lot of *in vitro* studies used only PRP which was not representative of an *in vivo* situation. The role of red cells, white cells, platelets and plasma must be taken into account.

Wautier: I think I agree. Most of the experiments of platelet aggregation was made in the past on PRP and many of the abnormalities which are observed or the effect of drugs have been missed by these techniques, so I think to use the platelet aggregation of the whole blood is a progress. And as you say you cannot predict everything with this test but it's a very simple test, it uses a very small amount of blood so it can be a screening test which can be useful to evaluate some drugs, for example, but not to predict thrombotic disorders.

Missirlis: When you say a platelet aggregation test to evaluate a device or a surface, do you mean to do the whole test with whole blood in the actual hemodynamic conditions that this device is going to be used for?

Ordinas: I believe that we could advance a little in the concept of platelet activation and, besides in the classical concept of measuring aggregation we should consider the importance of platelet released products. According to our present knowledge the interaction of platelets with any foreign surface results in a series of events that trigger the release of a variety of products. Thus, the indentification of one or more of these products could be an index of platelet activation. Could we decide here which one of the platelet-derived products is more indicative of this activation?

Cerletti: If there is a product to measure, that is thromboxane. It is very easy but is quite partial limited like measuring platelet aggregation. I think that different agonists should be tested because platelets can become unresponsive to one agonist but still keep aggregation to a different agonist. Another possibility which I don't know if it has been explored or not it is to measure the antigen on the platelet membrane, for instance the exposure of b-selectin should be an index of platelet activation occured. This is very experimental.

Wautier: We know that in platelet aggregation there should be some activation but it is something different. We can look at activation by measuring modification of platelet glycoprotein expression.

Ordinas: The current concepts of measurement of glycoprotein expression indicate that early appearance on platelet membrane of GMP140 is one of the best markers of platelet activation. As you well know, GMP140 is a membrane granule glycoprotein that is only expressed on platelet surface upon cell activation. Recent data obtained during extracorporeal circulation or even mechanical plasmapheresis or plateletpheresis indicates that platelets express GMP140 at very early stages of activation.

Kieffer: Since GMP140 is a glycoprotein present in the membrane of the intracellular platelet α granules, I am surprised that you can detect GMP140 on the surface of activated platelets without detecting the products that are known to be released from the α granules during platelet activation, such as PF4, βTG or TSP.

Ordinas: I cannot give you the specific reference but I recall a publication refering to the fact that GMP140 can be detected on platelet surface prior the release of any specific platelet protein such as βTG or PF4.

Wautier: I think you recall J. Georges' paper where he measured the expression of GP140 of platelets using flowcytometry and claimed in his paper that it was a very sensitive technique. I think that at the end it was not that easy to distinguish between the expression and the background. There is one point that is probably interesting to have the opinion of all the experts: what is best to detect platelet activation, which one you would recommend?

Davies: If you're looking for a best test it begs the question best for what? One answer being a circular argument saying this test is a good test because it correlates with all the other tests. And is the problem really that we don't have an end point to measure our test against? The only real test of platelet function is how does that platelet operate *in vivo* in its hemostatic role. We have touched on this area and we all agree that it's an extremely difficult thing to measure. So I think one of our problems with trying to design a "best test", and the reason that there has been such a plethora of claims for various tests of platelet function over the years, is that we can't really get at the end point that we want, which is a physiologically functionning platelet, because the only really good way that test of platelet function is whether it works in the circulation.

Wautier: If it's not possible to define the best test, could you possibly define the one which is not bad?

Davies: Most people in this field settle for doing a number of tests, because they accept there is not a single "best test". And I suspect it's going to be very difficult to devise a single "best test". There have been many new approaches: release of beta TG or PF4; release of serotonin; looking for degranulation of platelets or for expression of cell surface receptors, activation of GPIIb/IIIa or whatever. I don't think we have evidence that allows us to say that any of these tests is necessarily better than any other, because it comes back to the question better for what?

Ordinas: I agree with you but I still believe that the expression of GMP140 is the best test that we can use. Although, presently we must admit that there is no single test to fully evidence the stage of platelet activation. Perhaps combining two or three tests is the most convenient way to predict if there is any activation of platelets after blood has been in contact with a new biomaterial. We must remember that this is the aim of this meeting.

Davies: It depends more or less on the circumstances. If you are trying to evaluate a tube of some synthetic material to be used as a vascular graft in a circuit, I would suggest that if you measure beta TG (beta thromboglobulin) and you do it carefully it's a fairly good index of platelet interaction with the surface. But if you want to take platelets out of the system and look at the platelet to see how well its physiology is preserved, you are asking a slightly different question. And there I would have thought that some of the more recent tests look quite promising. I remember reading a paper on the use of monoclonal antibodies to the activated form of GPIIb/IIIa. That is a promising way of looking at the early stage of platelet activation.

Hanson: Measurements of platelet factor 4 and beta-thromboglobulin are useful but indirect indices of platelet activation. For example, in patients cardiopulmonary bypass produces elevated plasma levels of these markers and their depletion from the alpha-granules of platelets that continue to circulate. So in this and probably other settings of acute platelet activation these measurements may be useful. We also came to the conclusion based on these and other studies that measurements of dense granule release may not be useful since dense granule release is probably a fatal event for the platelet in most circumstances, despite some early literature to the contrary. With implanted chronic devices it may be useful to measure platelet survival or destruction although these tests reflect platelet reactions at all sites of vascular disease and not just platelet reactions with the prosthetic device. One can also perform Indium–111 platelet imaging to localize thrombus formation at the implant site. In a study like this in patients with aorto-bifemoral grafts, we determined that about 20% of platelet consumption was due to the graft, with the remaining 80% due to platelet reactions at other sites of vascular disease. Overall, both direct and indirect methods may be useful depending upon, among other things, whether devices are exposed acutely or implanted chronically.

Missirlis: As I mentioned before we have been measuring release of βTG in a flow experiment. That is we have tubes, we draw blood – it's an *in vitro* test – and we have a 10 min perfusion. So then we use the assay of Diagnostica Stago and we make measurements of the release of the amount of βTG. Now our experience is that it's a patient dependent, it is a nurse dependent, it is a syringe dependent result. At least these factors. But suppose that you can control these to a certain level, it's like using a filter to do away with noise. Then the next question arises: is it the constant shear stress that we apply useful for measuring these parameters in order to compare different materials? Or should we go to pulsatile flow? Or should we go to a closed circuit to recirculate platelets for some time? These are questions, and of course from an engineering point of view you can do all these things, but what is more relevant in terms of measuring this factor it is a questionmark for me. Can you suggest something?

Ordinas: This is an important aspect for you but I believe the basic problem is to find markers for early, not for late, platelet activation phenomena.

Missirlis: So you mean that one should have a more sensitive test to check some damage to the platelet but not enough to induce release. Is that the idea?

Hanson: I like very much the idea of looking for platelet membrane changes by flow cytometry, a concept that has been discussed for some years. However, I've only seen good documentation in older studies in patients on cardiopulmonary bypass, and in the analysis of blood effluent from bleeding time incisions. In such cases you may see alterations in glycoprotein IIb/IIIa, expression of GMP 140, and formation of platelet microparticles. Another marker may be platelet-associated Factor V. In our hands, these tests have been somewhat insensitive in a number of clinical situations in which you might expect platelet activation. Thus this approach may not be particularly useful in some settings, as is also suggested by the fact that there are not more compelling reports in the recent literature.

Kieffer: The fact that it is very difficult to visualize activated platelets with probes interacting with surface-expressed activation markers suggests that activated platelets might be rapidly sequestered and eliminated from the circulation.

Ordinas: I am not sure that flow cytometry to check glycoprotein expression has been used in studies of the interaction of platelets with foreign surfaces. What I know is that it has been used in patient under extracorporeal circulation and we have personal experience in patients undergoing hemodialysis.

Kieffer: These are extreme clinical conditions. It is certainly far more difficult to monitor platelet activation in patients at a prethrombotic stage.

Ordinas: No I do not imply that this technique should be used as a clinical diagnosis system what I want to say is that it should be applied to the study of the interaction of platelets with foreign surfaces.

Mulvihill: *in vitro* techniques could be interesting, for example fluorescent microscopy experiments. This method has been around for some while with the group of Feuerstein and there you can look at individual platelets arriving and detaching or forming aggregates, you are not looking blind. It strikes me as a very sensitive method which enables one to see in real time what is happening at a surface. Over a relatively short time we can see changes taking place. Some surfaces favour the formation of aggregates which then leave, while others favour monolayer formation. There are points for and against, but perhaps as an *in vitro* test if we want to look closely at surfaces it's not such a bad idea.

Missirlis: But these are washed platelets with a fluorescence probe attached.

Mulvihill: Platelets are not washed, they are fluorescently marked in whole blood. Admittedly there are problems with the markers and some authors have found for instance activated platelets, the extent of activation depending on the wavelength of fluorescent excitation. There are traps and artefacts in all these methods, this is true. However, if you compare a number of different surfaces by screening under the same conditions with the same platelets, such techniques may be of value.

Ordinas: The advantage of this type of experimental system is that due to the fact that you need a small amount of blood, it can be easily modified depending on the results of the experiment.

Wautier: Everybody agrees that we have several tests to detect platelet activation. The question is what is the more reliable, the more sensitive, the cheaper, the easiest to perform, so I think we have several questions and possibly it's not that easy to have a simple answer. When you have a lab which is very good in the radiolabelled platelets the easiest way to look at is to label the platelets and to look in the system. When you have a flowcytometry system which is working every day it's very simple to use this technique, or when you are measuring betathromboglobulin twice a week it's not also a big problem. Some of the tests are more easy to do in some labs and other in other labs. But Dr. Davies told us there is not real gold standard. I'm sure of this, but do you think that platelets survival and platelet deposition measured by the actual technique like Indium labeling is one of the techniques which gave the better credit or not?

Davies: Well, I don't know as much about this as Steve Hanson, but my experience of platelet labelling and trying to detect reliably platelet deposition on grafts and angioplasty sites in man is that the margin of error is quite large. I think measuring these things reproducibly in that way is difficult. And because we found it so difficult to get reproducible, quantitative, data we stopped doing it.

14. Biological tests for evaluating platelet biomaterial interaction

Davies: I see its attractions and I think theoretically it has a lot to commend it. Again, my experience doing platelet survival in rabbits and platelet survival with indium, chromium and aspirin labelling in man, is that there is quite a bit of individual variation. The problem with platelet survival is that you need to do quite a few to get a reliable estimate, and it is time consuming, and though not technically difficult, it is an awkward sort of process. So I have reservations about platelet survival. My view about platelet survival is supported by the fact that few groups now publish on platelet survival. It's possibly only groups like yours [Steve Hanson's] who have 20 years experience that feel comfortable with the technique, so I wouldn't see platelet survival as a front runner if we are trying to look for the best tests.

Hanson: Platelet survival reflects all normal and pathological mechanisms of platelet utilization in the body. To see a significant shortening in platelet survival you may need a significant injury. For example, angioplasty or endarterectomy may not be sufficient. One setting where platelet survival combined with platelet imaging may be useful is the vascular graft. While it may be difficult to quantitatively image small vessels or intracardiac thrombi due to the blood background radioactivity, imaging of aorto-femoral grafts can be reliably performed. In this setting you can derive quantitative information about rates of platelet deposition and the platelet residence time. Since this analysis requires steady-state rates of platelet arrival and removal from the graft, perhaps the only setting in which platelet survival may be useful is with established grafts that are actively thrombogenic.

Davies: Yes I'm sure that's right. You need a big artificial surface, you need some big injury in the circulation that's causing a lot of platelet deposition. Do you have any data that relate either platelet survival, or extensive platelet deposition on big Dacron grafts in man, to graft survival time, which is the ultimate test?

Hanson: To date we have only compared Dacron grafts and aneurysms. This study was published in *Arteriosclerosis*, 1990. While we haven't compared different types of grafts the method would be appropriate to do so.

Davies: But that isn't quite the point I was getting at. If you could say to me that you have done studies looking at platelet imaging and platelet survival

Y. F. Missirlis and J.-L. Wautier (eds.), The Role of Platelets in Blood-Biomaterial Interactions, 181–198.

and in those patients you found shorter platelet survival, and heavy platelet uptake onto the graft, and that those grafts don't survive as well functionally, then I would be convinced.

Hanson: We haven't followed these patients long-term to see if there are any differences in outcomes. While it might be argued that better grafts should show less platelet consumption and fewer embolic complications, we have not established such a correlation directly.

Davies: This is the difficulty, isn't it? A reasonably good aortic Dacron graft in steady-state, which has been put in by a competent surgeon, is going to last for 10–12 years and the patients frequently die of something else before graft failure. So, in that context it's really very difficult to say whether one sort of graft material is better than another. Because if they are done with technical skill, in that situation i.e. a large bore graft in a large artery grafts last for a very long time.

Hanson: The published study with established steady-state grafts may be largely of theoretical interest since it would be difficult to correlate with clinical outcomes. Of more practical interest would be to look at the platelet embolic shower that occurs immediately after graft placement. This certainly occurs in animal models, and may also account for occasional but serious episodes of lower limb ischemia that occur in man post-operatively.

Thus this early embolic phenomenon, which is probably important, may well be related to graft type and could rather easily be assessed by platelet imaging.

Ordinas: At this point we must consider if we have the biomerial ready to be studied for its reactivity towards circulating blood which system should be the most appropriate. We could define what kind of animal model we want to use.

Missirlis: I wish to come back to the previous point and ask the following: have all the markers for platelet activation been looked and checked after contact with surfaces? Is it possible, for example, small ions like calcium, which plays a role in most metabolic processes, to be a marker of more calcium inside or outside as an indication of activation or not?

Ordinas: I really do not know. It may be due to patent policy the companies that make artificial materials do not supply all the necessary information.

Missirlis: The question actually was if you make one or two tests, say βTG or PF4, is it enough or is it better to use other markers which are useful?

Wautier: We discussed about several aspects of platelet activation. We spoke first about what is the membrane modification. If we want to cover all the modifications of the platelet. I think it would be probably useful to look at this level first by studying the modifications of GPIIb/IIIa or GPM/140. Second the factors which are released from the platelets: PF4, Btg or TxB2. And in human situation there is an excellent correlation between TxB2 and Btg. So I guess we can use most of these but not all of these but one of these which is a marker of the intracellular release. We can use radiolabeled platelets. This has been done by J. P. Cazenave a long time ago to look if there is an interaction with some device with the platelets. And that you can quantify the amount of radioactivity which is associated to the biomaterial and in this condition evaluate the interaction between the material and the platelet. But I think that is probably not enough and that we'll switch to Tony and to the morphology. With radioactivity you don't know if it is one aggregate or many platelets sitting on a large surface so you need something more.

Mulvihill: I think we all agree that you must use a range of tests for different applications, for instance, bTG to measure platelet secretion, or thromboxane to follow platelet metabolism and the cyclooxygenase pathways. Since everything happens simultaneously, if you are comparing a range of tests, platelet imaging is probably one of the best. If you are looking for a cheaper animal model than the baboon or the dog, we have found that the rat, although not close to the human being as a species type, is nevertheless a small, inexpensive animal, easy to produce in large numbers and useful for screening tests. You can obtain a sufficient number of animals to perform good screening tests. We have established extracorporeal shunts in rats similar to those in baboons. Now we are trying to set up an Indium platelet imaging test to look at implants of different vascular materials in the rat, possibly after a preliminary radioscreening test *in vitro* to eliminate materials which are clearly very poor. The others will then be tested in the animal model. The only problem is that with this type of radiolabelling technique you cannot distinguish between aggregates, clusters and individual platelets. You measure platelet accumulation or deposition.

Ordinas: Of course, the more tests we perform the more blood we need.

Davies: You made a comment about measuring platelet associated factor V, which you rather threw away. Could you say any more about this?

Hanson: By flow cytometry, a monoclonal antibody specific for platelet-associated factor Va has been a very sensitive marker for platelet activation, particularly in patients with acute stroke.

Davies: Why do you think that is?

Ordinas: Have you published this information?

Hanson: This is not published.

Wautier: That is in favour of your idea that there is expression of the coagulation or so. The presence of the activated factor V on the surface of the platelets is in favour of the activation of the coagulation cascade at the same time of the other activation.

Hanson: Yes. There are questions as to where factor Va binds and how much paltelet activation is required for binding. These data might suggest that factor Va binding is an early step in the coagulation process that might require relatively little platelet activation, perhaps less than required to activate GP IIb/IIIa.

Davies: Do we know whether the platelets have to be activated to bind factor Va? Whatever activation it is.

Hanson: I'm not sure of that.

Wautier: Have you measured all the markers of the coagulation cascade activation like FI-FII proteolytic fragments or thrombin-antithrombin complexes?

Hanson: We have measured all of the conventional plasma markers. Certainly in the animal models they can all be elevated. In particular, the fibrinopeptide A level seems to be good marker.

Davies: I suspect that there are not major differences in what many of these tests are telling us. I think the reason why we have so many tests is because we can't be quite sure what it is that we are trying to measure, so we hope that some new test will prove to be more sensitive than the previous ones. But more sensitive for what? Or we hope some test would be better than the others but better for what?

Wautier: There was a recent report in Florence last week by R. Rosenberg. He has injected in man a very little amount of TNF and found that only this very sensitive test were modified in terms of the evidence of coagulation activation while the classical tests were completely normal.

Davies: What do you mean by the classical test?

Wautier: Well, for example FPA was not modified.

Davies: Well, one of the Dutch groups has published on this too. I think it was in association with them.

Ordinas: I think that at this moment we have more or less finished the possible tests necessary for proving the platelet activation phenomena. Maybe it would be interesting now to focus the discussion on possible tests to prove some kind of coagulation activation produced by a new biomaterial. In the past years many tests have been proposed such as D-dimer, FPA etc. so why don't we now move to this part of the discussion.

Davies: What you want to do with an *in vitro* test is to screen out the things that look so unpromising that it's not worth while to take it any further. Surely to do that you don't need to over-elaborate the technology? If you put a material *in vitro* into a test system, which causes a brisk rise in beta TG and the platelets, when you take out a sample, won't aggregate, and if you look at them under electron microscopy and there are not any alpha granules left, you know that the material isn't very promising. Or at least you know with a high degree of reliability that it's not a very promising material. We can't absolutely conclude that.

Hanson: Do we know that a platelet can degranulate *in vitro* and continue to circulate? This would argue that there are sublethal or non-adhesive encounters with biomaterials, or that adherent platelets detach and circulate. Perhaps the platelet changes are more sensitive than trying to assess coagulation-related events which are inhibited by anticoagulants in the *in vitro* studies. It would be of interest to look at the nature of the platelet-surface encounters microscopically, or indirectly using a radioisotopic label. Also, we might look at the number density of adherent platelets, the release of platelet-specific proteins, and changes in platelet count. Platelet membrane changes by flow cytometry could also be important. Beyond that, there isn't much I can recommend.

Missirlis: Even in this aspect the literature that we have looked at is confusing. People use sometimes one type of anticoagulant others use no anticoagulant, some use a loop system or different hemodynamics. Now we all know that each of these factors affects what we are going to measure. Besides there is the standardization aspect. How much to standardise? Who is going to say what? Who is going to say it? I mean we really had big problems as outsiders to know whether what we measure is compatible to something else that has been already published.

Wautier: I think at that point we have quite an agreement about the tests that could be applied to detect activation of platelets. I think that we have quite not a consensus but not far from that. So I think that's a good point. Possibly two years ago we would have a different discussion. It has become more clear at that point. Well the problem if blood is anticoagulated or not or which anticoagulant is used this is another question. So we cannot discuss all the questions at the same time but I think this would be useful. The first point is that there are some tests which are a little new, possibly more fashionable but it has to be proven to be as good as the tests that have been used before and I think for at least for a screening test it is quite clear. I will, myself, just make a little comment. I think it would be probably a little unclever not to look at coagulation since people told you that at *in vivo* situation coagulation starts to be activated. So for the future I would recommend to look at coagulation and at platelet agreggation.

Hanson: You could reduce the anticoagulant concentration to allow some thrombin to form.

Mulvihill: We found in our *ex vivo* test that if we had too much heparin anticoagulant we could not detect any FPA generation at all, but if we reduced the heparin level from about two units down to 0.15 units per ml there would be a little FPA formation. It was difficult to obtain steady and reproducible heparin concentrations, this is true. However, I think if you lower the anticoagulant level to a point where you have a sort of minimum anticoagulation what you see is a certain amount of thrombin generation. From our experience of trying to work *in vitro* with no anticoagulant at all, considering the lack of reproducibility of the results from taking blood from different donors and perfusing capillaries within a ten minute interval, we finally abandoned the idea. You have now obtained better results than we did, but at the time we went back to using an anticoagulant. Then I have one question : what do you think of hirudin as a possible anticoagulant? It does not affect platelets and it blocks thrombin. Until recently the price was prohibitive, but now the new recombinant hirudins have become available they are coming to be accepted as anticoagulants. Is there anyone here who has had experience with hirudin?

Hanson: Yes, we've studied hirudin in animal models.

Davies: It's difficult to get concentrations of hirudin where you get just a little bit of activation.

Mulvihill: We have found this too.

Ordinas: I would like to make a point at this moment. The perfusion model proposed by Sakariassen using a flat chamber and drawing native blood directly from the vein is probably the best technique to study the process of coagulation activation because in this system no anticoagulant is used. However, for doing studies with new biomaterials and checking possible coagulation activation the use of anticoagulated blood will permit longer experiments and I think that from a clinical point of view the use of hirudin will probably be the best anticoagulant because you still have calcium in the system and calcium is very important as you know. In the past many discussions have been generated about the use of citrate in experimental models so now that in the near future we will have the possiblity to use recombinant hirudin I think that it will be the best anticoagulant to use.

Wautier: I want just to make a point which is quite funny about the history of citrate. It's something which I read in the book of my son that the blood coagulation started when the blood was exposed to the air. I was a little surprised and I did not understand why they wrote that. I discovered it by reading old books until 1878. So people thought that the blood clot occured just because it was in contact with the air in the atmosphere. And things changed when one gentleman or two perhaps at the same time found that when you add citrate the blood did not coagulate at all even in presence of air, oxygen or everything. So I agree that citrate is an old one but we have to realise that before citrate was discovered we did not know that calcium was important for coagulation.

Ordinas: I agree with that. Are there any more comments about anticoagulants?

Missirlis: Is there one hirudin or many? I have heard of many hirudins.

Hanson: The recombinant hirudin we've studied lacks a sulphate group as compared to natural hirudin. There are also hirudin analogs.

Davies: There are subtle differences between hirudins from different species of leeches, as I understand it. I think there are minor modifications. I think there are three hirudins, at least.

Wautier: You mean natural hirudins?

Davies: Yes, but I'm not a hurudin expert.

Mulvihill: There are slight changes in sequence and conformation but the performance as an anticoagulant seems to remain comparable.

Davies: The big problem with this approach, and I'm sure we all recognise it, is that we are making the assumption that we can wipe out thrombin and just think about platelets and surfaces in isolation. And is that really a sensible way to approach it?

You [to Steve Hanson] have published a paper with something in the title saying that thrombin is the most important.

Hanson: If you abolish thrombin completely you may markedly impair platelet reactions and their accumulation on surfaces. So it may be better to employ minimal anticoagulation with heparin, hirudin, or other agents and let some thrombin form. Another possibility is to use a factor Xa inhibitor.

in vivo, these inhibitors preserve platelet function better than the direct antithrombins, and with less bleeding, perhaps because some thrombin is still formed. As far as I know, factor Xa inhibitors have not been studied with biomaterials *in vitro*, but it might be interesting to do this and compare, for example, with results obtained using heparin and hirudin.

Wautier: I think there is one point we have to recall : that in the Baumgartner system the first which has been published in 1972 and in which they were studying the adhesion of platelets to subendothelium system. They use 3.4% citrate which is lower than the usual amount which is 4%. An when you use 4% you have no platelet deposition. And there is no real good explanation for that. It could be that you need a minimal coagulation activation to have a real deposition. So if we switch from citrate which is the old one to a new thrombin specific inhibitor, we could possibly completely modify the system.

Mulvihill: I think one important point might be that platelets require calcium for their metabolism, so if you lower the citrate concentration of the medium the platelet activity could be affected. By adding less citrate you may leave a sufficient external calcium level for platelets to achieve a more normal metabolism.

Wautier: But when you are looking at platelet aggregation in PRP you can use citrate 4%. So it makes a big difference without adding calcium. So you can have perfect platelet function in PRP with 4% citrate while in the Baumgartner system with 4% citrate you don't have platelet adhesion to subendothelium. That's the difference.

Davies: The main advantage is that we have a long experience of it [citrate] and we know by altering the concentration that you can allow platelet function to proceed and you can allow coagulation to proceed. My concern is that if thrombin is a major mediator of platelet reactions with all sorts of artificial materials in the circulation, as we all suspect it is, then there is not much point in doing *in vitro* assesments in a system in which you've abolished thrombin generation. So I think there is quite a bit to be said for going on using citrate as the primary anticoagulant. You may get some interesting additional information by using hirudin, but I would be a little reluctant to suggest that we should switch from citrate, which is what most people use, to hirudin, without having thought carefully what the implications of that might be.

Wautier: Further more the anticoagulant which is used for blood transfusion is mainly citrate.

Ordinas: Well, what we are trying to do is to make a maximal approach to what happens *in vivo*. You have mentioned the Baumgartner perfusion technique. We have some experience with this technique and if you use citrate as an anticoagulant you are able to see the different types of interaction of platelets with the subendothelium such as contact, spread, adhesion and aggregation, but never formation of fibrin. But you know that in humans the generation of thrombin and the formation of fibrin is very important. That is why since recently, with the use of this perfusion technique we have been using low molecular weight heparin as an anticoagulant, and with this system we are able to modulate the formation of fibrin in perfusion. We think that now with this new approach we are closer to studying what happens *in vivo.*

Missirlis: So, you are coming to the conclusion that a low level of anticoagulant, either citrate or hirudin, is going to allow for a synergistic effect of the coagulation system to the platelet activation. And this level, does it depend on the application that you want, or do you know what this level is?

Hanson: We don't know, but it would be a straightforward study to reduce the anticoagulation and see how this affects the results.

Mulvihill: Yes, I think it depends on the application. For instance, if you are working with heparin or low molecular weight heparin, when you are doing *in vitro* tests and wish to conserve your blood in the laboratory for a certain period of time, you will tend to add a little more anticoagulant. In our *ex vivo* tests, we standardised the anticoagulant level by pretesting all our volunteers for their sensitivity to heparin and adjusting the amount added to the blood in the dialyser inflow so as to double the activated partial thromboplastin time (APTT). The amount of heparin required to double the basal APTT varied from about 0.12–0.18 units per ml according to the subject. Hence we took the coagulation test as a guide to standardise the level of anticoagulation. In our particular application, we found that this heparin concentration allowed us to detect a little FPA formation at the outlet of the dialysers. Likewise bTG and activation of platelets. However, this was in a particular instance and it might be necessary to design each experiment specifically with respect to anticoagulation.

Davies: Do you think there is any point in considering the use of defibrinating enzymes? At least that allows you to generate thrombin and look at the thrombin effect on platelets.

Hanson: The enzymes can be pretty messy. If we could characterize all the fragments produced, and their effects on platelets, it might be of interest to study defibrinogenated blood. I don't think we can recommend this at the present time.

Davies: Is everybody happy that the semi-synthetic, low molecular weight, heparins have no effect on platelets?

Wautier: They have some effect. It is published.

Ordinas: In our experience we recently found thrombocytopenia in a patient treated with low molecular weight heparin.

Davies: But the thrombocytopenia that you get with heparins is immune-mediated thrombocytopenia. It's not necessarily quite the same thing, is it?

Ordinas: We think that this thrombocytopenia was related with low molecular weight heparin because when the heparin was discontinued the platelet count went up.

Wautier: Apparently but there is no real serious publication comparing the incidence of the apparently occuring thrombocytopenia using standard heparin versus low molecular weight heparin. But in terms of *in vitro* modification of platelet function by low molecular weight heparin and standard heparin it's quite similar.

Davies: So, you're left with the same problem, that there is a poorly quantified direct effect of heparin-like molecules on platelets, the basis of which we don't understand.

Mulvihill: I think you cause a lesser degree of platelet activation with the low molecular weight molecules. I have done one or two *in vitro* perfusion tests using a standard heparin anticoagulant in parallel with a low molecular weight heparin and I observed the platelet adhesion to be reduced in the case of the low molecular weight product, about 20–30% lower.

Ordinas: I think that maybe now we can go on. I think that we agree that when the new biomaterial is ready it must be checked in an animal model. We know there are several different animal models with the most popular being man. Perhaps we could discuss which animal model would be best before its testing in humans.

Davies: How often can you use your baboons? Can you use them once a day, can you put in a new shunt once a week?

Hanson: The chronic shunt typically lasts for months, and we can interpose devices or materials on a daily basis as long as the daily individual studies don't perturb the hemostatic system too much. For example, we wouldn't want to change the platelet count significantly between studies.

Davies: And they don't get infection from the catheters and so on?

Missirlis: How many labs use baboons, apart from you and Seattle?

Hanson: Four, I believe. But it's a complicated and expensive system that I would not recommend for general use.

Davies: I don't think you need to be too frightened of the competition. You can't feed baboons at 5 dollars a day.

Hanson: One question to consider with all models is whether evaluating materials in idealized configurations or simple geometries predicts their performance when constructed into actual devices. If the simple tests are not predictive, this would preclude the use of small animals for testing materials used in large devices, since we would have to evaluate the actual device.

Missirlis: Well, what is your opinion about that. I tend to think that the device is the ...

Hanson: My opinion is that if we must have reliable performance data, then actual devices should be evaluated in their intended usage configuration, and preferably in a primate. Such testing is probably more likely to be predictive of results in man, although we haven't clearly proven this. At the same time, simpler testing would be very valuable so we need to continue working in this area to hopefully establish correlations between the results of different tests in different animal species, and in man. At the moment we may have no predictive *in vitro* tests for devices, although its clear that the material composition of devices is important. For some devices we may not even have good animal models although the performance of vascular grafts may correlate reasonably well between some animals and man.

Davies: Would you say from your experience that if a graft tends to behave reasonably well in one or more animal species then it's likely to perform reasonably well in humans?

Hanson: Yes. For example, based on a great deal of animal and clinical data there is a consensus that Teflon grafts, such as Gore-Tex, perform better than Dacron grafts in small caliber applications such as below the knee bypass. However, there may not be many examples like this where animal and clinical studies are in reasonable accord.

Davies: Probably because not many comparisons have been done. I don't think there is any reason to favor one animal over another on a scientific basis. So one really is left going for practicallity and economics again.

Hanson: Important differences between animals have been documented. For example, a number of years ago platelet deposition onto artificial surfaces under flow conditions was compared for dogs, pigs, primates and humans. Results varied by orders of magnitude between species with primates and humans giving the most similar values. However, this was an idealized test and there have been few such comparisons. So I agree that it's still a matter of practicality to the extent that we don't have a lot of data for recommending one species over another.

Missirlis: So a rat that is cheap is it a useful model?

Hanson: At this point, perhaps. But in the future the rat may prove to be less useful than other species for predicting the performance of materials used in man. We will need more data to establish which is the case.

Mulvihill: One of the disadvantages of the rat is that if you wish to test a large device this is difficult in a small animal. We hope to be able to evaluate dialysers in rats but by reducing their size, scaling them down by one in 25 or even smaller according to the size of the animal model. There again we may encounter scaling problems.

Missirlis: The scaling problems in terms of construction can be solved, but I'm now wondering about suturing very small vessels, for example if you have to test grafts.

Mulvihill: If you have a good surgeon this can be done. Our surgeon in the beginning did have some problems with suturing and found it very difficult to reproduce his results. However, with practice he discovered that the grafts were patent for longer times, 12 hr as compared to initially 2 hr for a graft without any collagen or thrombogenic insertion. Results were also more reproducible. It therefore takes practice when the vessels are small and technically can be difficult but is still feasible.

Davies: Maybe what you need to make successful grafts is a very old, experienced surgeon.

Ordinas: I think that once we have decided on an animal model then we have to decide the type of tests that would be appropriate to evaluate whether the graft is functioning correctly.

Hanson: I think radioisotope imaging will continue to be useful, as will measurements of activation products of platelets and coagulation. We will also need endpoints including patency rates, frequency of complications, and evaluation of explants microscopically and macroscopically.

Missirlis: Regarding the microscopic examination. When you fix red cells to see them at SEM you don't expect to do much damage to the cell. Is it the same with platelets? I mean when you see a spread platelet, or the nice picture you showed us, is it the actual case just before you fix the platelet? Or glutaraldehyde does alter it?

Ordinas: I think that with the current techniques which are faster than those used in the past, we are sure that what is seen in the images is what actually occurs. I agree with Dr. Hanson that a picture is only a confirmation of what has happened within the graft and it is always nice to show a picture demonstrating a thrombi inside of a graft with red cells and platelets trapped in a fibrin net.

Hanson: To do this by radioisotope imaging could be problematic because of the high platelet background associated with tissue injury at the surgical sites.

Mulvihill: People used to think it worthwhile to look at platelet deposition after the first short period of implantation of a graft in a human being, did they not?

Hanson: With a graft platelet survival and imaging may be useful but perhaps not with other devices such as, for example, the current generation of heart valves which are less thrombogenic than older style valves. With valves and other devices you may have to rely on indirect markers and outcome events.

Davies: We've done some work looking at hemostatic functions actually during surgical operations and I'm not surprised you've got a huge release of PF4, FPA and so on. So the degree of activation of the hemostatic mechanism you get in during a fairly staight forward abdominal operation is such that I'm sure it's days before you can reliably conclude it has released products.

Hanson: It may be more important to look at endpoints of clinical consequence such as embolization, ischemia, myocardial infarction, and occlusion, as may occur with grafts, stents, aortic balloon pumps, and so forth.

Missirlis: Coming back to the questions of what are the limitations of those measurements; you put a radiolabel marker or an antibody or fluorescence what do you do to the platelet? I mean how do you change its properties? I remember N. Kieffer said that when you bind fibrinogen on a ligand a signal is transmitted from the outside to the cytoplasm. Did I understand well? What does that mean?

Kieffer: When fibrinogen interacts with GPIIb-IIIa, this binding does indeed generate intracellular signals. For example, fibrinogen induces a conformational change of GPIIb-IIIa which can be monitored by specific monoclonal antibodies. Fibrinogen/GPIIb-IIIa interaction does also induce tyrosine phosphorylation of platelet proteins and the synthesis of specific metabolites of the phosphatidylinositol pathway, such as phosphatidyl 4,5 bisphosphate.

Missirlis: Maybe I was not very clear. When you put antibodies to test for example in flow cytometry some early activation do you already change the platelet that you wish to study? This is my question.

Kieffer: Yes, if you use metabolically active platelets in your experiments, or let us call these platelets living cells, then antibody binding can induce changes in platelets. In fact, it depends on whether you use metabolically active or inactive platelets. Let us consider one example. You want to study the reorganisation of platelet membrane receptors during platelet adhesion using monlonal antibodies as probes to visualize the receptors. If you incubate living adherent platelets with an antibody and keep the experiment at 37°C, the antibody by itself will induce artefactual receptor clustering. However, if you perform your adhesion experiment at 37°C, and then incubate your adherent platelets with the antibody at 4°C, you will be able to visualize the adhesion-dependent redistribution of the receptors.

Wautier: But it's a fact, it's not an artefact.

Davies: It comes back to this old question of how you decide what the physiological state of the platelet is. If you can show that it will aggregate well to standard agonists, if you know what you are doing, (for example, it is possible to mess up radiolabeling and damage platelets very badly) but if you know what you are doing, the platelets will aggregate following radiolabelling. It is impossible to say they will survive normally, because the only measurements of survival we have use radiolabeled cells, so it's a circular argument. But they appear to perform well using *in vitro* tests. So I think you have to accept that as soon as you take a platelet out of the circulation, and start doing things with it, you will modify it to a certain extent. A platelet is such a reactive cell, it's almost inconceivable that you can label it without altering its function is some way, but you just have to live with that.

Missirlis: So it's the Heisenberg's uncertainty principle somehow, when you want to measure a property you already interfere with the measurements.

Many people: Yes.

Hanson: Not necessarily. We have good data to suggest that radiolabelling of platelets may not significantly affect their survival or function. For example, platelets are typically labelled with Chromium–51 or Indium–111, both of which require *in vitro* manipulations to separate platelets from the blood, or they can be labeled *in vitro* or *in vivo* with no blood manipulation using 14-C-serotonin which is taken up into platelet dense granules. We have done this in humans and animals and have compared the platelet survival data obtained with these methods.

If you take platelets which have been subject to all the manipulations of

Chromium–51 or Indium–111 labelling, and concurrently label them with 14-C-serotonin *in vitro*, you get the same serotonin platelet survival as if you had just incubated the serotonin with whole blood *in vitro* and reinfused, or injected it intravenously and allowed it to be spontaneously taken up *in vivo* by circulating platelets with no platelet manipulation. While you have to be very careful, of course, since you can injure platelets *in vitro*, this result argues that these procedures do not necessarily shorten platelet survival. In animals, you can also show that platelet labelling does not significantly affect platelet function by challenging the animals with injections of agents such as ADP, thrombin, collagen, etc., or by exposing highly thrombogenic surfaces to flowing blood in a recirculation loop. In all cases the reduction in total circulating platelet count, which comprises all labelled plus unlabelled platelets, is equivalent to the reduction in platelet radioactivity associated with those platelets, typically 5–10% of the total platelet count, which are radiolabelled. This argues that the labelled and unlabelled platelets function in an indistinguishable manner. Thus, while it does take a lot of experience and careful technique, platelet radiolabelling can work very well.

Davies: It's almost certain the way you are looking at it. We are deceiving ourselves if we think that unlabelled platelets are similar to ...

Hanson: *In vitro*, platelets may be dysfunctional after labelling. After infusion *in vivo*, they tend to recover normal platelet functions.

Ordinas: Many years ago with the use of the Baumgartner perfusion technique we were able to show that labelling platelets with either chromium or indium the platelets labelled with indium functioned better than those labelled with chromium.

Missirlis: Is this generally accepted? We have to use chromium in Patras because we import it from abroad and indium having a short half life, is more expensive for us, so we are trying to label platelets for *in vitro* experiments with chromium. Do we make a serious mistake by doing that?

Hanson: Not necessarily, but you have to use higher concentrations of Chromium than Indium, and perhaps additional washing steps, because the labelling efficiency is not as great. You might also use a beta emitter such as tritiated or Carbon–14 serotonin.

Mulvihill: One of the reasons why people use Indium is that it is a more powerful emitter and therefore provides a more sensitive probe. Indium emission is of higher intensity than Chromium emission. When looking for thrombosis in a clinical situation, practicians use Indium labelled rather than Chromium labelled platelets because they give a stronger signal under the gamma camera and you can detect venous thrombosis more easily. Thus apart from possible platelet damage, the preference for Indium is also to obtain higher sensitivity.

Ordinas: Now I would like to make a question to the experts because it is hard for me to understand the procedure followed to arrive to having a tube or a material which can be used in humans which we must work with to see whether it interacts with platelets or activates coagulation.

Missirlis: The tubes we used in our measurements were made by a company, Rehau is the name, under a Eurobiomat contract, as Dr. Lemm said, in order to have the same batch. So all the laboratories collaborating had the same material, not from different batches. They were extruded-came out like spagetti. Many people can take a PE tube, for example, and then can change the inner surface by chromic acid or some other acid that can induce changes in the inner surface and then put another material onto this already formed tube by dipping it into a solution. You can do many modifications with physical techniques, with radiofrequency, glow discharge, you can change the properties of the inner surface by many different physicochemical techniques. Or you can have your own material, like W. Lemm has PU solution from-I think it takes a long time to make tubes by dipping a metal rod for example and then let it dry and then dip it more to have a variable thickness. So there are different ways. Now we are involved in a project with an Italian group in Siena and they are making new materials and we want to make tubes out of that. But that material is not extrudable so we don't know how to make the tubes that we wish to have. Most probably we'll use a dipping technique in order to get out tubes. Other people have more experience.

Lemm: But the easiest way is to use a polyurethane tube and to coat the inner surface.

Davies: Then it comes back the issue that you raised earlier, whether you can totally ignore what the rest of the tube is made from and whether the inner lining is all that really matters.

Hanson: It is probably the outermost surface layers that affect platelet adhesion and the earliest blood reactions.

Missirlis: Mechanical properties are very important. It seems that the literature shows now, especially for grafts, that impedance matching should be there otherwise in the long run it would create problems.

Hanson: Has that been shown convincingly in a study with compliant grafts?

Missirlis: Well, Lyman's recent paper indicated that. He had materials of different impedance in an artificial model and showed that, with generating the same flow through these different impedance pairs, the amount of the deposition of platelets and fibrinogen, I think, was different because of the impedance difference.

Hanson: Where did that paper appear?

Missirlis: In the journal of Biomechanics, I think it was 2 months ago. And I think there is some work in Liverpool by D. Annice and T. How where they have some data on that.

Hanson: I thought the Annis graft had been abandoned at one point.

Missirlis: Well they are reworking on that, I think.

Hanson: Are they?

Missirlis: Yes.

Ordinas: If there are no more comments we can go on to the final conclusions.

Wautier: I did not prepare any special conclusions but I can try to say a few words. First I want to thank and to congratulate Yannis Missirlis for the organisation of this meeting. I think the atmosphere was very pleasant and the seting is marvellous. I think we've known most of us before coming but after such a meeting I think we'll leave from Samos being all friends. So I think it was possibly not the only goal of this meeting but that has been achieved anyway. Besides that I think we covered many points about the interaction between platelets and biomaterials and how it's relevant to the problem of health in general. We discussed about transfusion and what could be the future. We're very satisfied with most of the products at the present time but there is some improvement which can be made. In materials that can be implanted in human, I think we have made a lot of progress in defining what are the tests we can apply to try to select first tests for screening before testing these materials in animals or in humans. So I think we could have, after these days, a more clear view of what could be done to help the people who create new materials or to tell them what is the requirement we have for a new material which could be more compatible in the human body in the future. And I think it is an area which would be developed in the future first, because we can hope that the traffic accidents will reduce so the potential donors for organs will reduce too. That's something we have to keep in mind. And besides that that the age of the population is also increasing and we will need to be able to replace some of the organs which will be altered just by aging. So I'm quite confident in the future of biomaterials and I think our meeting is probably promising for the development of this area. For the last but not the least point we are people here from different countries of Europe and the States and I think it is very important that as people do in the United States, realize that they can communicate, and they can also communicate between Europe and the States. It's a small channel ! I think it is not so expensive and it is not longer to go from the side to the other. We have a good model in the States where people can communicate and can move from one state to the other and we hope that it's time for Europe to do the same.

Missirlis: I enriched myself these two days not only from meeting all of you but also from the scientific point of view. I think it's going to take me some time to digest what was said here, but I think it was useful to have people from different backgrounds both scientific and also practical. In that sense the EEC project EUROBIOMAT, whose coordinator is W. Lemm has been doing a great job in organising such symposia where free discussion and exchange of ideas is coming and maybe some of us got a few ideas that we can put them to work later on. So I really wish to thank W. Lemm for giving us this opportunity to meet here.

Lemm: The purpose of this workshop was to join experts, both the hematologists and the chemical engineers whose task it is to develop better hemocompatible biomaterials. We met at the interface of both disciplines and some unpredictable events happened as it really happens in nature as well. Because of our different educational background we had some difficulties to understand each other. I had problems to get familiar with the problems of the hematologists and their technical terms and I suppose *vice versa.* In my opinion, such interdisciplinary expect meetings are of extraordinary importance in order to provide each other with a profound knowledge and a deeper awareness of interfacial problems. I confess that during these two days I learned more than studying books for weeks.

I would like to express my thanks to Prof. Wautier for taking over the scientific organisation without hesitation. I also thank Prof. Missirlis for the local organisation and arrangements and finally Prof. Hanson, for coming and sharing his experiences with us.

Index of names

Index of subjects